REVERSING
CHRONIC
PAIN

REVERSING CHRONIC PAIN

A 10-Point All-Natural PLAN FOR Lasting Relief

MAGGIE PHILLIPS

Foreword by Peter A. Levine

North Atlantic Books
Berkeley, California

Published by
North Atlantic Books   Illustrations by Andrea Bryck
P.O. Box 12327   Cover design © Ayelet Maida, A/M Studios
Berkeley, California 94712   Book design by Brad Greene

Printed in the United States of America

Reversing Chronic Pain: A 10-Point All-Natural Plan for Lasting Relief is sponsored by the Society for the Study of Native Arts and Sciences, a nonprofit educational corporation whose goals are to develop an educational and crosscultural perspective linking various scientific, social, and artistic fields; to nurture a holistic view of arts, sciences, humanities, and healing; and to publish and distribute literature on the relationship of mind, body, and nature.

North Atlantic Books' publications are available through most bookstores. For further information, call 800-733-3000 or visit our website at www.northatlanticbooks.com.

Library of Congress Cataloging-in-Publication Data

Phillips, Maggie.
    Reversing chronic pain : a 10-point all-natural plan for lasting relief / by Maggie Phillips ; foreword by Peter A. Levine.
        p. cm.
    Summary: "A guide to how the body's wisdom can help resolve its pain, this book presents 10 effective skills that provide readers with tools to join their body's resources with mind, spirit, and heart, tipping the scales of their somatic experience away from unrelenting pain toward balance, comfort, and, eventually, pleasure and vitality"—Provided by publisher.
    Includes bibliographical references and index.
    ISBN-13: 978-1-55643-676-5
    ISBN-10: 1-55643-676-9
1. Chronic pain—Alternative treatment. I. Title.
    RB127.P493 2007
    616'.0472—dc22
                                                        2007020153
                                                        CIP

2 3 4 5 6 7 8 9 SHERIDAN 14 13 12 11 10 09 08

Acknowledgments

I am deeply grateful to the many people who have made this book possible. First and foremost, I want to thank my clients whose openness to experimenting with alternative treatment methods and courage to teach me the unique dynamics of both their suffering and resiliency have been deeply moving and indispensable catalysts for expanding my own learning.

Many colleagues have contributed to the ideas and methods contained in *Reversing Chronic Pain*. To thank properly all who have encouraged, taught, treated, suggested, guided, and mentored me over the years would require a volume in itself. I hope you know who you are. Each of you has contributed to my growth more than I can express.

Finally, I want to thank the supportive circle of friends and family members who have believed in me throughout the chapters of my life: My parents and brother who first taught me about the healing power of love, the members of my spiritual community who inspire me to practice what I teach, and most of all, Andrea and Casey, who are my guides to joy in each day. The blessings that all of you bring instill the faith and strength to keep reaching for miracles that release and resolve pain in every new moment.

Table of Contents

CHAPTER TWO

Feel: Turn On Your Body's Built-In Pain Regulation System . . . 25

CHAPTER FIVE

Mindfulness: Fill Your Mind
with the Wisdom of Each Moment . . . 85

CHAPTER EIGHT

Pendulate: Heal the Trauma—Pain Connection . . . 145

CHAPTER NINE

Love: Embrace the Heart of Your Pain . . . 165

Foreword

The unfortunate truth is that at some time in our lives most of us will be affected by chronic pain. Right now more than a hundred million people suffer from pain in the United States alone. The fortunate truth, however, is that resolving even entrenched chronic pain can often be surprisingly simple. This is the great lesson of *Reversing Chronic Pain* by Maggie Phillips, my friend and colleague of more than twenty-five years.

There are two grand killers of life: the twin sisters of pain and fear. Indeed, fear and pain feed on each other, keeping us immobilized and unable to engage in life. Based on her decades of work with trauma, as well as clinical hypnosis, imagery, energy psychology, and Somatic Experiencing®, Dr. Phillips has masterfully distilled what is essential for helping people overcome and heal their chronic pain and their fears of chronic pain. Her book is the result of more than thirty years of clinical experience and the development of a highly regarded and successful online pain program.

The vision of this book goes well beyond managing pain. Pain can be healed if we are willing to take the rich journey into a united body-mind. In drawing from her knowledge of Somatic Experiencing®, Maggie Phillips utilizes the understanding that (in the absence of a physical-medical cause) most chronic pain is generated by our bracing against certain physical sensations. We begin to fear these physical sensations and responses that were originally self-protective in nature, tightening up against them and causing them to become maladaptive. However, in doing so we actually create that which we fear the most—pain! As told by the Buddha some thousands of years ago, it is as though we are shot by one arrow and then shoot ourselves again (in the same place) with another.

In this book, Dr. Phillips helps the reader untangle the sensations, images, and thoughts that co-create the fearful dragon of pain. Once de-fanged and liberated, these very energies that were "locked up" in the belly of the beast (the "bracing" patterns of pain) are freed to live within us. Hence, this book not only helps to reduce or eliminate pain but also facilitates the transformation of the very way we live our lives. This extensive program supports and empowers the reader in moving from helplessness to feelings of hope, vitality, goodness, and well-being.

Dr. Phillips begins by suggesting that specific types of pain and their location in the body (whether from migraines, herniated spinal discs, fibromyalgia, chronic tendonitis, or from unresolved grief reactions) are not the real issue. The approach used to manage all pain successfully is relatively similar.

The key to resolving persistent pain, Dr. Phillips emphasizes, is being connected to one's body. This critical understanding is minimized in most books on pain, yet body awareness is simply one of the most potent methods for shifting pain. Most people in pain, understandably, either don't want to focus on the body in ways that can provide lasting change, or don't know how. In *Reversing Chronic Pain*, Dr. Phillips helps the reader reclaim the body self in a way that is gradual, safe, and effective in providing lasting pain relief.

The other important (and almost universally neglected) part of working with pain and with the mind-body partnership is the importance of trauma. Dr. Phillips notes that we encounter many situations that challenge our bodies to survive threat. These survival responses are stored in the brain and the rest of our physiology and become our blueprint for future self-protection. However, when unresolved, trauma forms the bedrock of chronic pain. The author helps readers untangle this web and free themselves from trauma's strangle grip.

Each chapter in this well-organized book presents a specific skill set for cultivating body awareness. Each skill set builds on the skills learned in previous sections. Readers are offered a "menu" of practice exercises that are designed to facilitate reconnection with the body-mind. Unique levels of readiness, interests, and needs are acknowledged and respected.

In addition, Dr. Phillips provides resources in many practical areas, including nutrition, gentle exercise and stretching, and various types of "bodywork" methods found in the reader's own community. If you are a sufferer of pain or have loved ones who are in pain, this is a book for all seasons. Read on and take a healing journey toward empowerment and wholeness.

— Peter A. Levine, PhD, author of *Healing Trauma: Restoring the Wisdom of Your Body*, *Waking the Tiger: Healing Trauma*, and *Trauma Through A Child's Eyes: Awakening the Ordinary Miracle of Healing*

Introduction

If you are reading this book, I imagine that you are in serious pain and/or that someone you love may be in pain. I want to welcome you to a program that has helped many people out of pain and which I believe offers that possibility for you.

In my twenty-five years as a psychologist working with clients who have struggled with pain conditions, I searched for a magic bullet that would be powerful enough to put an end to pain. While I have been fortunate to help many people move out of severe physical and emotional pain using a variety of helpful tools, I have not yet found that magic bullet, nor do I know anyone who has.

What I have learned about healing pain is deceptively simple: There is no single method that works for everyone. I offer an intensive, integrative program that teaches a set of highly portable skills, which can be easily learned and practiced anywhere so any person in pain can generate reliable interventions. Ultimately, what will work for *you* is not just what experts believe "should" solve the problem, but rather a self-customized plan built on *your* actual results.

What Does It Mean to Reverse Your Pain Condition?

When I work with someone in chronic pain, I work to find a strategy or combination of techniques that will—as quickly as possible—start to tip the scales away from a downward spiral of increasingly debilitating pain into a place of greater harmony, balance, and comfort. Often it can be challenging to find that tipping point,[1] but it is never impossible. And once the scales begin to tip against pain, additional methods can keep the momentum going in the direction of greater and greater freedom from the effects of pain.

Over the years, I have learned several important lessons about how to reverse the course of pain:

- Specific types of pain and their location in your body do not influence pain treatment as much as you might think. Although it's helpful to gain an understanding about the problem that may be causing your pain, the tools you use to manage it successfully will be similar to those used to treat other types of pain. So whether your pain is connected with migraines, herniated spinal discs, fibromyalgia, chronic tendonitis, or a grief reaction to loss (for example), the basic approach is the same.

- It's virtually impossible to resolve a persistent pain condition without being connected to your **body.** Although it certainly makes sense to involve the body when treating pain, most people in pain either don't want to focus on their bodies in ways that can provide lasting change, or don't know how. Body awareness is simply one of the most potent methods for shifting pain. If you are connected to all types of sensations, including pain, you will have a much better chance of finding permanent relief. The central focus of this book is helping you expand your body awareness and learn to use your body's natural resources to solve the puzzle of pain that lingers.

- Without guidance from your mind, your body can get lost in primitive, painful reactions. *Reversing Chronic Pain* will teach you to use your head to harness the wisdom and potential of your mind to work as a capable partner with your body so that you can reach your full potential for resolving pain and regaining full health.

- One important part of working with the mind-body partnership is to pay attention to **trauma.** Over our life span, we encounter many situations that challenge our bodies to survive threat. As with animals in the wild, our survival responses are activated by our brains and the rest of our physiology. What we learn from each survival experience becomes our blueprint for future self-protection.

Unlike animals in the wild, however, our body blueprints for survival are often interrupted. If we are threatened by assault, loss, or injury, our body responses may be acceptable during the crisis and immediately afterward, but if traumatic experiences are prolonged, we usually receive messages from those most affected by our reactions that we need to "get over it." Unfortunately, the body often cannot easily get over threat because the mind doesn't know how to work cooperatively with the body's natural reactions to trauma. Within our somatic experiences are clues for elegantly resolving pain patterns that are linked to our body's attempts to protect and survive.

- For each of us there is a tool or combination of tools that will help bring us to the "tipping point" to begin to reverse the pain cycle. Although I can't predict the most successful tools for any given person, I am confident that with creative exploration, persistence, and collaboration, the key can be found that will "unlock" the problem and begin to uncover the solution. This book provides an extensive array of keys to try. By the end, you will have learned to befriend your body and to teach your mind to work as your body's partner in seeking hope and eventually freedom from a life centered on pain.

Why We Need Another Pain Book

The success that my clients and I have found in reversing the course of stubborn pain conditions has led me to the belief that *every* path that effectively reverses pain leads through the body. Most people in pain understandably try to avoid their bodies in a vain attempt to avoid their pain. Many wrestle with the side effects of strong drugs that remove them from their bodies, further traumatizing them and ultimately creating more pain. Cutting off access to either the mind *or* the body creates more overwhelming stress and further disconnection from the vital resources that could end the reign of pain. It's hard to believe that so few of the many good books about treating pain teach the reader how to approach pain from the body's point of view, as well as from the mind's perspective. I have learned that it is absolutely *essential* to reopen the path often closed down through pain that leads us to mind-body connection, wholeness, and full engagement of our innate pain relievers.

This book offers a brief, intensive, integrated model that I have piloted with many people individually as well as in a group format. The method is centered on learning to experience your body as the ultimate healer in your recovery from pain by finding and using your body's natural resources, and by regulating its responses to traumatic experiences, including pain that persists even though the threat and danger have vanished.

I am happy to report that among the total number of people who worked with the program presented in this book, about 95% have improved; roughly 50% have dramatically reduced their reliance on prescription pain medications along with their pain levels; and about 15% have discontinued their regular use of prescription pain medications altogether while their pain remains at significantly lower and livable levels.

What to Expect from This Book

Each chapter presents a specific skill set related to body awareness and found to be important in reversing the course of chronic or persistent pain.[2] Each skill set builds on the skills learned in previous chapters. Practice exercises are designed to facilitate reconnection with your body and partnership with your mind. You are invited to sample what is appealing and appropriate in terms of your unique levels of readiness, interest, and need. Completing each exercise involves nothing more than practice, the willingness to set specific goals for recovery, and the ability to work independently while exploring and experimenting. Readers who are challenged in these areas can easily work through the material with assistance from a trained professional, such as a psychotherapist, or visit our website at www.maggiephillipsphd.com for supportive services.

Move at your own pace through the book, learning new strategies and reviewing familiar ones. The exercises are designed to stand alone and have been "field tested" by people in pain, many of whom found them helpful. It's likely that you will find at least a handful most effective in helping you toward the "tipping point" of your pain. It's very important that you learn to trust and stay with what works for you, and let go of what doesn't seem to work or feel right, rather than trying to prove that you can master every method contained in each chapter to "get the most out of" this book. Some exercises simply will not be right for where you are at this time, and that's OK. You can always consider trying those again in the future.

You are likely to benefit even more if you keep a pain notebook or journal that focuses on your experiences with this book. You can record your progress, questions, and discoveries as you go along. It's a good idea to skim through the material in each chapter first to pinpoint which sections and strategies you believe will have the most value so that you focus your attention on them. Then move through the chapter a second time with the intention to master those tools you have bookmarked on the first reading. Once you have begun to master one skill from each chapter, you can cast your net wider to consider other approaches or move on to another chapter.

Each chapter joins information and direct experience to provide ample possibilities for shifting pain by assembling a solid foundational building block. The function of each building block is to bring together resources of mind and body to achieve a specific type of *body awareness*. This term reflects the powerful combination of bringing mental, spiritual, and emotional awareness to body experience. The result is a 10-point pain program that interweaves elements of mindfulness, breath practice, creative imagery, self-suggestion, and somatic focusing to help you produce a personal pain protocol that brings *reliable* and lasting relief.

One way to organize your learning is to consider using each chapter to shift your pain one point on a 10-point rating scale, where 10 is intolerable, out of control suffering. Even if you start this book at a "10," by the time you finish, you may be at one or even zero.

I hope you will learn as much about being your own best teacher and healer as about how to treat your pain. Many people who have been in intense pain for more than a few months have been told what to do, and have been judged by others if they fail to complete or respond to the prescribed treatment. **You** are the final authority on what steps recommended in this book work or don't work. Discarding approaches that don't seem to work is as important as refining what does help you.

So start gently, and gradually build momentum. There is no race to run, only the adventure of learning with and from your body how to get out of debilitating pain, and how to live with greater clarity, comfort, and strength. As you work your way through this book, you will assemble a toolbox of life-changing strategies to guide you on the road to health and wholeness. I wish you well on the journey.

CHAPTER ONE

Be With Your Body and Breathe
The Reign of Pain Is Mainly in Your Brain

One of the most important principles related to reversing chronic pain involves the mind-body connection. Research has confirmed that pain experience is governed primarily by the brain and its varied states of awareness, as well as by other parts of the body.

The word "psychosomatic" reflects the fact that pain, as well as other symptoms of health imbalance, are governed both by the beliefs and moods of our "mind" experience as well as our body's physiology or somatic experience. Unfortunately, *psychosomatic* has become a dismissive term, and that can be misleading. When using this word to describe health situations where there may be some type of psychological conflict or issue that is being expressed in the body, many people have come to assume that psychosomatic symptoms are created by a person's mind when there is no "real" medical problem. This misunderstanding has led, in part, to the more recent use of the term "*mind-body connection*" to describe the rich interconnection between mind and body experiences.

The truth is, *all* sensation including pain is governed by the mind-body connection—as much by psychology as biology. Research has taught us, in fact, that the mind and body are intertwined even at the cellular level.[1] So although it is not actually possible to separate one from the other, distinctions within this book are made purely to give

1

us specific entry points into the mind-body process of healing. Throughout *Reversing Chronic Pain*, you will encounter tools designed to develop the "mental" ability to guide the body, as well as those used to refine your understanding of how your body communicates with your mind.

It is essential to establish a solid partnership between mind awareness and body experience that unifies all efforts to recover. We must learn to use our "heads" to help our bodies recover. In other words, we can't just treat the site of persistent pain in the body and expect to attain permanent healing. When people are not successful in reversing their pain conditions, I find that their minds are often urging their bodies to "try harder," push through pain, or hurry up and "get over it," while their bodies seem to be relaying messages of "I can't try any harder than I'm trying. You have to help me get out of this pain now!"

Yet the body's pain messages seem to be continually alarmist and hysterical—"I will always be in pain"; "there's no way out"; "it's hopeless to try"; and so on. Obviously this kind of conflict between "mind" and "body" makes it very difficult to respond to *any* method of healing. That's why one of the central messages of this book is to help you discover the powerful healing possibilities that exist when mind wisdom and body presence are aligned and working together.

What You Don't Know about Pain *Can* Hurt You!

If you have persistent, unresolved pain, you have probably been given a diagnosis and have some idea about what is causing your pain. Yet, ironically, what you've learned about the cause of your pain may yield few clues about how you can actually stop the pain and heal its wounds.

This first chapter discusses the natural partnership between mind and body that regulates your pain, and how you can participate actively in this process. You will learn skills that can help you make an immediate positive difference in your experience of pain. These serve as the foundation for a healing program that supports an experience of lasting relief for you.

It's a good idea to read this chapter twice. Skim it first to get a sense of its basic plan, and then move back through the material in a second pass, allowing enough time to master what you are reading. Remember, even though you may be acquiring several new skills throughout this chapter (depending on your needs), our overall goal is to help you tap the resources that are yours when you are present in your body. The good news is that the body is continually healing itself. If we learn how physical healing happens naturally, we can actually help this process along rather than unintentionally obstructing it.

How Pain Operates: The Automatic Gate System

What does it mean, exactly, when we say that pain is governed in important ways by the brain? To answer this question, we need to know something about the mechanics of pain. One of the best-known theories about pain was proposed in the early 1970s by two researchers, Ron Melzack and Patrick Wall. Melzack and Wall determined that pain is regulated by a gate system[2] in the spinal cord that receives pain impulses and transmits them to the brain.

Simply put, different types of nerve fibers located throughout the body are trained to transmit pain signals received from various sensory receptors to the spinal cord and brain. Once nerve impulses reach the brain, they are interpreted either as a threat, which generates anxiety and pain, or as more neutral sensations. So, the reason for this chapter's heading, "The Reign of Pain is Mainly in Your Brain," is to point out that the brain decides whether a particular sensation is dangerous and therefore painful.

The thalamus (located in the brain) serves as the "router," sending each signal received from the dorsal horn structure in the back of the spinal cord to three different brain sites. These include the sensory cortex, which registers physical sensations, the limbic or emotional center, and the thinking brain in the frontal cortex. Each of these areas has an influence on how we respond. Usual possibilities are that we can ignore the pain if positive competing experiences have beaten the pain signals to the gates; we can react and be flooded with pain if fear and stress have prompted the amygdala in the limbic emotional system to sound a serious alarm; or we can respond to the pain as information about our most important body needs, including the need to escape or survive a situation or stimulus that is threatening for us.

Pioneer pain researchers Melzack and Wall discovered that certain circumstances "open the pain gates" governed by the dorsal horn in the back of the spinal cord so that pain messages are relayed without interruption to the pain centers in the brain, and that other experiences "close the gates" and stop the pain signals from ever reaching the brain. One of the main objectives in this book is to teach you multiple ways of controlling the pain gates to reduce the amount of pain that passes through.

Types of Pain

Pain is usually considered *acute* when you have had an accident or injury to your body that results in predictable patterns of significant pain that require treatment. *Chronic* or *persistent* pain continues even when healing has taken place and the pain is no longer serving a beneficial purpose. The goal of professionals who work with you is to help you manage the intense impact of the pain you feel so that its initial protective function will gradually lessen and become unnecessary.

There are several physical mechanics to consider in understanding how pain operates. *Muscle pain* is one of the most common types of pain. Muscle spasms occur when the body contracts all muscles near a painful area in an attempt to "splint" the injury and immobilize it. Spasms can become prolonged because the pain they generate can result in further spasm, thus creating a vicious circle of pain–spasm–pain–spasm. So, what began as a beneficial protective device goes awry when the body becomes stuck in the mode of sounding the alarm.

Prolonged muscle spasms can sometimes cause chronic musculoskeletal pain, especially back and neck pain. Another problem caused by muscle spasm is *referred pain*, which is pain in a different location from that of the spasm. For example, repetitive pain in the right arm, such as that resulting from carpal tunnel syndrome, may trigger pain in such "strange" places as the left shoulder or the thoracic mid-back area, because of a chain reaction through what are known as *myofascial trigger points*.

Trigger points are created by injuries, straining of muscles, and various types of stress reactions. They can be activated by additional strain or stress. Upon activation, they create spasm in the muscles that surround the trigger point, which then creates a pain cycle that may not be localized in the area of the trigger point. Later in this book, you will learn ways of finding and working with your own trigger points.

A second general type of pain is *nerve pain*, which may occur when nerves are injured but can also occur when damaged nerves later regenerate imperfectly, causing new nerves to fire randomly and in error, so that they send pain signals to the brain even in the absence of pain.

To a certain extent, all pain is nerve pain, because most pain begins with peripheral nerve endings that pick up pain signals. Sensory nerves receive the sensory signals related to body movement and pressure as well as tissue injury. Injury to any of these nerves is believed to cause neuropathy, which results from injury to the axon, the inner information pathway of the nerve cell, or to the myelin sheath that protects the nerve cell.[3]

Good News from the Gate

Thanks to the research of Melzack and Wall, we know that dull pain or neutral or positive sensory messages travel much faster through the nervous system than painful sensations. Soothing sensations such as direct pressure and the touch of massage travel up to seven times faster, for example, than sharp or burning pain.[4] This means that if soothing as well as painful sensations enter the dorsal horn at the same time, the faster, more pleasant sensation will prevail, blocking transmission of the slower, painful one. This fact brings good news for the pain patient! One of the main ways of reversing the course of pain is to find what creates consistently reliable body experiences that compete successfully with pain.

For example, many people who are absorbed in a good book, movie, or play or a pleasant family interaction do not experience even intense pain. Others might use a cream or ointment containing capsaicin,[5] the active ingredient in hot cayenne pepper, as a topical remedy to block pain by creating a heat sensation that competes with pain and often wins. *Think about what you use now in your daily life that creates immediate or rapid sensation to override your pain.* Your pain blocker may be as simple as using ice or heat or a topical analgesic such as "Icy Hot" (which contains capsaicin), or as complex as using pain technology like acupuncture needles, biofeedback, or a TENS (transcutaneous electrical nerve stimulation) unit.

Keeping a focus on body or somatic experience is essential in learning to regulate and reduce your pain. To achieve this goal, it is important that you know what already blocks your pain most reliably.

Recognize How Your Body and Mind Are Already Blocking Pain

Take a moment to think about what is already working for you and *list your top five current pain blockers*. To come up with a response, you may want to review your typical daily routine even as recent as today or yesterday. Notice where you feel better, have more energy, or can be more active. Identify the behaviors that precede and follow these times. Are there any surprises?

↤ SAM

Here's an example. Sam first came to me complaining of migraine headaches. When we looked together at what his mind-body system was already doing to block pain, at first he could not identify anything, saying, "It feels like I have the pain twenty-four hours per day. It's *always* there."

"It may be always there," I said, "but when are you *least* aware of it?"

After thinking for a while, Sam was able to come up with three blockers. And after a week or two more, he developed a complete list:

1. When there's an important meeting at work and I'm really into it, I'm not aware of the pain.
2. When I'm in the shower in the morning, I don't feel the pain very much.
3. I can get away from the pain while I'm listening to a mindfulness CD.
4. When I go to a baseball game with my son or watch a sports event on TV with him, the pain disappears.
5. Sometimes when I go for a bike ride, I get focused on nature and that disconnects me from pain for a little while.

What's YOUR list of pain blockers? You might want to list them in your pain notebook, or right here on this page, or perhaps write them on a bookmark for this chapter that can remind you of important points.

Now that you've identified your top five pain blockers, use them consciously and consistently every day for the first week or so that you are reading this book. Write them on post-its as reminders in certain places, or keep a list on your calendar or in your pain notebook. What do you notice after you have activated this intention for a few days?

Specific Techniques for Closing the Gates on Pain

So far we have mentioned one important way of closing the pain gates: by stimulating sensations that compete with and override pain. This closes the gates in the dorsal horn by blocking pain from traveling to the brain. An example is the use of capsaicin, discussed above.

In addition to the pain signals traveling up to the brain from the spinal cord, the brain is also sending return chemical messages down to the spinal cord. Some of these chemical messages, such as the endorphins created by aerobic exercise, can block out the pain completely.

Thus a second way to close the gates is to help stimulate the brain to generate powerful positive chemicals to counteract the impact of pain sensations that have already been allowed through the gates. A good example is the use of different types of breathing practices, meditation, guided imagery, and self-suggestion that can turn on powerful mechanisms in the nervous system and brain, and which can transform pain sensations you may be already feeling into more neutral and even positive somatic experiences. We will be working intensively with these methods through the rest of this book.

A third way to close the gates on pain is to regulate *inflammation,* a contributor to many kinds of pain. When pain messages receive a "green light" from the dorsal horn and are registered in the thalamus, the amygdala in the brain's emotional (limbic) center sends alarm signals back down to the tissues, muscles, and other parts of the body. One such alarm turns on increased blood flow to help repair any damage. However, some of the extra blood may leak out of the blood vessels and cause heat, stiffness, soreness, and swelling.

Usually inflammation resolves when an injury heals, but as pain persists and becomes more permanently encoded in the nervous system, inflammation can continue to cause soreness. Other sources of inflammation include diet and the side effects of many medications used to treat pain. When misdirected inflammation becomes systemic, diseases such as arthritis, myocarditis, asthma, nephritis, colitis, and other "-itis" conditions can result. In addition, surgery often damages muscle and tissue, which can create scar tissue. A buildup of scar tissue can then become a constant irritant to surrounding tissue, fascia, and muscles, also contributing to inflammation.

There are many ways of fighting inflammation.[6] Three of the best are strategic use of ice; anti-inflammatory, nonprescription drugs such as ibuprofen in appropriate doses; and the intake of certain foods or supplements. If you haven't already, please talk to your pain professional about how inflammation may be contributing to your pain, and what to do about it.

Finally, a fourth general way to close the gates on pain involves impacting four neurotransmitters that interact between the spinal cord, the brain, and the rest of the nervous system. These neurotransmitters have significant roles in spreading negative pain messages, which often keep pain persistent and chronic. They are *serotonin, GABA, substance P,* and *dopamine.*[7] These chemicals are influenced by genetics and also by the depression cycles that often accompany persistent pain. Certain foods,[8] herbal remedies, medications, exercise programs, and massage or other types of healing touch can help regulate these four chemicals responsible for trans-mitting sensory information between nerve cells.

Although the use of supplements is controversial because many are not approved by the FDA, you may find that some of them are helpful in reducing your pain. *Remember: It is always important to consult your prescribing doctor before taking any supplements or homeopathic remedies.* A list of twenty top pain supplements is included in the appendix.

In addition to these methods, there are many other strategies that can help to close the pain gates. These include medications, rest and adequate sleep, acupuncture and other energy methods, meditation, and positive thoughts. We will be addressing all of the above in the coming chapters.

What Opens the Gates to Increase Pain:	What Closes the Gates to Decrease Pain:
Lack of sleep or disrupted sleep	Good rest and sleep
Stress	Relaxation and self-treatment
Anxiety and fear about pain levels	Confidence in using tools to block or interrupt pain
Ruminating about pain	Distraction from pain
Depression	Increased serotonin
Deficit of endorphins	Enhanced endorphins through exercise & other experiences
Nutrients that increase inflammation	Nutrients that decrease inflammation
Repeated trauma to the pain area	Techniques to relieve pain areas; avoidance of unnecessary surgery or invasive medical procedures
Boredom, inactivity, too much activity	Increased interest in daily activities; appropriate activity level

Expose Your Myths about Pain
That May Block Recovery

Persistent pain that has not been responding for more than six months to usual treatments is usually referred to as *chronic*. This means that the initial cause of the pain has resolved, but the pain that persists has become a primary, chronic condition in itself. At this point, treatment is focused on the general pain condition rather than on the back strain or arm tendonitis (as examples) that first triggered the pain.

So, in addition to understanding the mechanics of pain, it is helpful to explore myths about pain that may be embedded in what you have been told by professionals and other people (or read somewhere), and to discover what is erroneous in what you are telling yourself without realizing it. "Debunking" or dismantling these myths yields additional choices in approaching everyday pain. Such myths are disempowering because they are false beliefs that restrict your ability to make clear choices about the abundant resources that surround you.

Several common myths about pain follow. *Take a moment as you read along to notice which ones elicit any type of internal reaction in your body. These are the ones that you might want to pay more attention to as being more "alive" or true for you. Consider what you can do (or are already doing) to counteract each myth.*

MYTH 1: I have to learn to live with the pain. There's nothing more that can be done. This belief is usually reinforced by professionals who have reached the limits of what *they* know to recommend to you, and it also implies that you are too demanding or perhaps not complying fully with the treatment methods that have been offered. This statement speaks of the dangers of despair, hopelessness, and helplessness in approaching pain.

Remember that there are literally hundreds of pain relief methods, and more are being developed every day. At least some of them will be unknown to every practitioner. One or more of them may be just right for you. If you sense that your treating professional is not responsive to your quest for permanent relief, maybe it's time to find another one who will be an active partner in your search. Feed your hope, not your negativity.

MYTH 2: There is *one* special doctor, medication, high-tech intervention, surgery, etc., that will stop my pain. This belief can be particularly hard to put to rest. We so want to find that magic bullet! Usually there is NO one approach that will resolve your pain. Persistent pain is so complex, there is no one root or underlying cause. Consequently, there is usually no one approach that will resolve it. Most experts believe that a combination of traditional and alternative methods is necessary to shift your pain gradually from center stage in your life to a less intrusive, more remote position.

If you have followed the evolution of treatment for HIV and AIDS, you may have heard about the "AIDS cocktail,"[9] developed after several years of effort to find the most potent medication to slow down the disease and relieve its debilitating symptoms. Ultimately, what worked best was a combination of medications that was more potent than any single medication because of the principle of synergy—the whole is greater than the sum of its parts. With the AIDS cocktail, it was the combination of ingredients that gave the most potency to each component. This is similar to what happens in cooking. The final product consists of much more than the eggs, sugar, flour, milk, and other separate ingredients that are blended together. The most effective pain treatment, in my experience, involves a combination of several approaches, each of which works optimally for a given person.

MYTH 3: I'm not getting better because I am not motivated enough (or smart enough, strong enough, etc.) to follow all the suggestions that have been given to me. I really dislike this one—if there are hundreds of pain interventions and each one involves multiple sets of directions ... well, you do the math! This myth conveys an overwhelming and impossible expectation. It is more likely that you are not following directives because they either aren't helping you significantly to warrant your energy, or because the pacing of the approach is not right for you.

Any given intervention can be broken down into smaller steps, and each one of those may be more appealing and approachable than the total assignment or exercise. If you are not responding, take a deep breath and find loving compassion for yourself and trust that there may be a very good reason why the approach may not be working for you.

MYTH 4: Everyone else is getting better faster than I am. When I hear this from my clients, I tell them that many pain clinics, physicians, and specialists have a "bell curve" that they use to plan treatment. (You may remember from math class that a bell curve is the statistical distribution of numbers so that about 68% of the members of any group fall in a "normal" range.) It's important to remember that you may be in a different place from the "norm" at any given point in your recovery—for example, maybe your response to treatment is in the 1–2% at either end (i.e., much faster or slower).

In fact, if you have persistent pain, by definition there are complex factors that may have delayed your progress. Many of these include external events over which you may have no control such as work or family crises or changes in your healthcare coverage. A far better approach than competing with other pain patients around you is to compete only with yourself by asking, "Am I moving in a positive forward direction even though my progress is slow? Am I in a significantly better place than I was a year ago?"

MYTH 5: Unless I get rid of this pain, my life is not worth living. The despair and frustration reflected in this statement is certainly understandable. Yet even if you can reduce significantly the intensity and/or frequency of your pain, it is highly likely that you will have some remaining traces of pain in the form of periodic flare-ups or certain sensations that remind you of the vulnerability in parts of your body. So it's important to ask yourself, "How will I live if my pain does not disappear completely?"

To dismantle this myth, we need to distinguish between pain and suffering. The pain itself is a particular set of body and mind reactions, while suffering is the hurt of pain—the impact of your pain reactions on your life. Suffering can be addressed and greatly reduced so that physical pain is no longer a nuisance and no longer controls your quality of life. You will learn many ways to reduce both pain and suffering in this book.

The Top Strategies for Pain Relief [10]

Now that you're beginning to understand the mechanics of pain and to dismantle some of your own myths about it, let's explore what the latest research shows to be the most effective ways to resolve pain conditions.

Virtually every book or article I have read on pain emphasizes the following components (though not necessarily in this order):

1. **Body-focused therapy.** This includes massage, physical therapy, Pilates, acupuncture, yoga, Reiki, and various kinds of exercise programs that are supervised by a professional, at least in the beginning. You may also want to use an approach like Somatic Experiencing® to focus on trauma in the body. In my experience,

it is essential to connect directly with your body's felt sense of pain in order to reverse the course of any given pain condition.

2. **Medication and medical treatment.** It is important not to dismiss the significance of pain medications. At certain times in your recovery cycle, well-chosen medication may be the only intervention powerful enough to break certain patterns such as intense, extreme-pain cycles, pain-induced depressions, and sleep disruption that prevents healing from taking place.

   Many people who are prescribed pain medication dislike the side effects they encounter, or they are afraid of the risk of drug dependency, and so resist taking medication. This is more than understandable when side effects compromise daily quality of life. Yet medication cannot work effectively *unless* you are taking the proper dosage for the right length of time (which may be longer than you would like) so that the drug can be useful in the ways it was designed to be. Such medications might include antidepressants, anti-anxiety compounds, and sleep aids, as well as pain relief medications.

   Other medical treatments to consider include nerve blocks, trigger point injections, and electrical and ultrasound stimulation. For the right person and situation, these can be invaluable.

   "Combination therapy" as explored in this book may make your use of pain medications more efficient. Many of my clients, as they assemble tools that harness the full power of the mind-body partnership, find that they begin to rely less on medication, or to use it strategically so that it brings more of the results they want. So, consult with professionals to make sure that you are not either overmedicating or undermedicating your pain.

3. **Nutritional therapy and supplements.** This factor is often ignored and yet is one of the most crucial in offering a relatively easy way to make a powerful positive impact on the pain system. Some foods, including sugar and simple carbohydrates that metabolize

into sugar, can provoke pain flare-ups. Conversely, there are other foods such as fish that can help reduce inflammation and pain.

You will benefit from learning about nutrients like antioxidants that relieve inflammation and boost the immune system. You will also benefit from an emphasis on nutrients and/or medications that increase serotonin,[11] which is depleted by pain. Serotonin blocks our perceptions of pain, stabilizes negative emotions and moods that increase pain, and helps to regulate sleep and the fight/flight/freeze response in the nervous system. You may want to consult a good nutritionist experienced in working with pain and other persistent health problems who can help you evaluate your nutritional needs. Herbalists, homeopaths, and acupuncturists can also be of help.

4. **Regulating daily rhythms.** This strategy involves regulating your daily schedule so that you have the right balance of activity and rest, social interaction and quiet, energy-giving activities as well as those that deplete energy. My program invites you to shift your daily rhythms so that they support pain reduction.

Perhaps, as some of my clients have done, you'll need to view the time you require daily to focus on recovery from pain as *self-treatment* rather than "rest" or "recuperation," since these are terms that may ignite your own judgments and those of others. Deciding to focus on effective self-treatment might allow you to place greater priority on healing in your everyday life and help you interrupt your pain cycle. *Pause right now and think for a moment. What would really give you permission to put greater emphasis on healing at this point in your life?*

Set Goals That Lead to Rapid Relief

It is common for people in persistent or chronic pain to feel unfocused, overwhelmed, and unsuccessful. Yet if you set *one self-treatment goal each week, you* will begin to bring organization to your day and deliver observable results by the end of each chapter. Even if it feels awkward at first, setting goals that are right for where you are with your pain can be one of the powerful tools to help you find lasting relief.

Start by choosing specific treatment strategies from each of the five categories presented above that can help you reach your personal *pain goals*. Now is a good time to start your *pain diary* or *pain notebook* that is used only for the purpose of tracking your goals and progress as you work through this book.

Before you go any further, set a goal to focus your reading of this chapter. As you go back through the chapter to work with the techniques and the exercises, keep this goal in mind to center your attention.

Make sure that your goal is:
- measurable (you can tell when you've accomplished it),
- realistic (you know you can do it),
- behavioral (involves specific behaviors, actions, or steps), and
- desirable (important to you *now* at this particular time).[12]

If you want to lower your pain levels as your goal, how will you know when you've done so? "I want to feel better," for example, is not a clear goal. "I want to reduce my arthritis pain from an average of 8 out of 10 on a pain scale[13] to a daily average of 7.5 or lower using one of the breathing methods presented in this chapter" *is* a goal that meets these criteria. If your goal includes a reduction of pain, be sure to measure your pain levels every day. Use a scale of 0 (no pain) to 10 (maximum pain). Give your pain a number to reflect its intensity. You can do this several times a day and average the numbers to get your pain number for the day.

Keep the 10-point scale in mind as you work your way through each chapter. Consider this: If you are able to use the tools in each chapter enough to lower your pain consistently by only one point, by the time you finish this book, your pain will be close to zero, or at least at livable levels!

If you feel stuck or are having trouble clarifying a goal, you might check with friends, partners, or loved ones who know about your pain problem. It could be helpful to hear what their goals are for you. Even if you don't agree, their feedback might help you clarify what you feel ready to tackle.

Be sure to record your goal for this first chapter in your pain notebook or another convenient location to help you keep focused before you go on. Another idea is to make a special bookmark to remind you of your goal as you work your way through each chapter, and on which to summarize your discoveries.

Why Breathing Is the Greatest Inspiration

We start with the breath because it is fully accessible and completely portable, and because shifting the breath can immediately turn on the restorative, calming branch of the nervous system known as the parasympathetic system. One simple, conscious breath can help close the pain gates, stimulate the brain to create pain-relieving chemicals (such as endorphins), and balance the fight/flight/freeze reactions responsible for transmission of pain through the nervous system.

Many pain patients breathe with short, shallow breaths in response to pain and its stresses. Unfortunately, this kind of breathing tends to maintain stress and to increase anxiety, which also increases sensitivity to pain. Many pain experts recommend that breathing exercises be done several times during the day and especially when pain levels rise or spike. One reason why deeper, calming breathing alone can lower pain is that it shifts brain wave frequencies from the beta waves that usually accompany the hurt of pain to more calming alpha frequencies.[14]

Most people in severe pain tend to hold their breath as part of the body's constricted, freezing response. Many also become shallow breathers because of the anxiety, tension, and stress that accompany persistent pain. Stress and anxiety can cause tension in the abdominal area, which means that the diaphragm is not free to expand and contract fully during the breathing cycle. This kind of constriction can prevent sufficient oxygen from moving through your system to cleanse toxins and promote complete healing.

Breathing practice is deceptively simple. Although most of us know something about how essential it is, we often dismiss the way we breathe as "not that important." The truth is, learning how to breathe properly, especially at times of increased pain and stress, is the *single* most important skill you can learn. Awareness of *one* breath cycle in and out connects you to the mind-body partnership, turns on the relaxation response,[15] and turns off the fight/flight response.

The first step toward using your breath for healing pain is to practice *natural* diaphragmatic breathing. Diaphragmatic breathing is helpful in two ways: First, it helps to remove carbon dioxide from your blood while creating oxygen, an important source of energy. Second, this type of breathing helps to stimulate your internal organs for overall health.

Basic diaphragmatic breathing involves learning to move your diaphragm more fully as you breathe rather than keeping your breathing high in your chest. The exercise that follows represents a common approach to this type of breathing.

Exercise: **Diaphragmatic Breathing**

When you are practicing diaphragmatic breathing, it helps to lie down on your back on the floor, couch, or bed. Place your hands just above your stomach. When you breathe in slowly through your nose (count from 1 to 5 seconds), you should feel your hand moving. As you breathe out slowly through your mouth (again counting 1–5 seconds), you will experience a calm, relaxed feeling without even trying. A good time to practice diaphragmatic breathing for 3–5 minutes is while you are engaged in an undemanding activity, such as listening to music or watching TV. Also practice at times when you become more aware of your pain or when it seems to suddenly increase, or spike. It is hard to be in pain when you are breathing through your diaphragm, because expanded breathing helps to counter the tightening and freezing related to pain.

SUMMARY: This first chapter introduced the gate theory of pain and some strategies that both open and close the gates on pain. In addition to what you already know that either increases or stops your pain, you read about the importance of examining common myths about pain and considering the top evidence-based strategies that resolve pain and reverse its course. We also discussed the AIDS cocktail approach to pain, which holds that effective pain treatment often is found in a *combination* of the most potent pain interventions for any given individual. In the next nine chapters, you will have an opportunity to identify specific treatment ingredients for your pain equation that, ideally, result in persistent relief from pain and begin to reverse the course of your symptoms. You will start now by using this chapter and the exercise below to help you move toward your first goal. Keep your goal in mind as you complete Skill #1 of the exercises.

Body Awareness Skill #1

**Be with Your Body and BREATHE:
Your Breath Holds the Key to the Mind-Body Partnership**

You may have already used breathing exercises elsewhere in your treatment. This exercise gives you a chance to learn some new breathing approaches to add even more choices. Find the method below that seems to create the most comfort and feeling of well-being, or feel free to add another approach from a different source (such as yoga or meditation) that appeals to you. You can also substitute simple diaphragmatic breathing, which you just practiced, if that feels best to you.

If you have structural limitations related to breathing such as severe asthma, pulmonary disease, or cracked ribs, *do not stress* about the mechanics of the breathing methods described here. What's most important is a simple focus on your breath. That alone will bring many of the benefits you are seeking.

With this exercise, as with all others to follow, please give yourself full permission to modify these directions in *any* way that works for you. What's important is that you give yourself a good experience, not that you follow the directions accurately!

1. First, simply **practice one or more of the breathing exercises**[16] **below.** Follow the directions (or modify them so that you can) as you explore how to use the breath to create calm, cleansing, or comforting sensations.

a. **Calming breath.** *Sitting or lying comfortably, inhale through your nose only until your abdomen is filled with air, then allow the air to fill your lungs. Hold the breath briefly and then exhale slowly through your nose, first emptying the lungs and then the abdomen. It may help to put one hand on your diaphragm just above your belly button and the other on your chest to better feel these changes. Complete five of these breath cycles. Breathe normally for a minute or so and then repeat five calming breaths again. When you feel relaxed enough, repeat the cycle, this time imagining that your breath is flowing into the area of pain or discomfort in your body. Feel this area expanding as the breath expands.*

b. **Foursquare breathing** *involves making a square in your breath cycle. Inhale for a count of four, hold for a count of four, exhale for four,* *and hold again for four. Repeat for a total of ten full breath cycles. When you are ready, imagine that your breath is flowing into the area of pain or discomfort in your body. Feel this area expanding as your breath expands.*

c. **Circular breathing.** *With this approach, imagine that your breath flows up one side of your body as you inhale and goes down the other side of your body as you exhale. It is usually more effective to link breathing in with the less painful side of your body, and breathing out with the more painful side. For example, if your right shoulder and neck are usually in pain, imagine breathing up the left side of your body, visiting places of relative comfort, and breathing out the right side of your body, imagining that your breath touches areas of discomfort and pain. If this is not effective, reverse the order, breathing up the painful side of the body, and exhaling down the more comfortable side. Repeat this for five to ten breath cycles.*

d. **Purifying breath.** *Imagine that your body is surrounded by light, healing sound, color, or healing presence (any one of these or a combination that works for you). As you inhale, imagine that you are sending that light into your lungs and abdomen and then throughout the rest of your body. As you exhale, imagine what is being expelled from your body—perhaps tension or constriction, sensations of discomfort, stress, pain, worry, or feelings of emotional pain. Repeat this process for five to ten breath cycles.*

2. **Breathe and block the pain.** Now use the breathing exercise that seems to work or feel best and combine this with some of the pain blockers you are already using. That is, as you repeat the breathing exercise this time, review the things that block your pain, whether they be reading novels by your favorite author, eating chocolate, watching mindless TV programs, or playing with a pet or your children or grandchildren. It may help you to use the list of your top five pain blockers from earlier in this chapter and even add to it.

No activities are too silly or "unhealthy" to include. As you breathe through the cycles, add a focus on these options that is linked to comfort. Notice what differences take place as you add this focus.

3. **Find a body-safe place or sanctuary.** Believe it or not, even though you may feel that all of your body is at the mercy of pain, there is *always* a place inside you that is unaffected by pain. Here is one way to find it:

Repeat the breathing exercise that you have chosen once more. This time on the first breath cycle, focus on creating comforting/calming/expansive sensations in the area of pain by repeating step one above. Then for the rest of the cycles, find or create a refuge in your body where you can curl up like a cat in the sun to rest, retreat from, and escape the pain. Keep your focus there for the remaining breath cycles.

Before you leave this chapter, have you been able to decrease your pain levels by half a point? One point? What could you add to make this possible? Do you need more practice? Sometimes it helps to review the chapter yet again, revisiting the steps that most helped you and refining your skills before you move on to the next chapter.

CHAPTER TWO

Feel
Turn On Your Body's Built-In Pain Regulation System

When we are in pain, we want to be *anywhere* other than where we are. It is extremely difficult to accept persistent pain, regardless of the circumstances. We are acutely aware of our setbacks and disappointments, of the exhaustion and helplessness we feel, and of the despair about what to do when we are blocked from making progress despite all our best efforts. Yet the old axiom is true: What you resist persists. Acceptance of your current pain rhythms is essential for forward progress. Without acceptance, the fight with pain can end up as an impossible battle that you will keep losing against yourself.

Why Wait for the Magic Bullet?

The common denominator for people in pain is the longing for relief and a *permanent* end to pain. We hold out hope for a magic solution in the form of a medication, new treatment technology, or a spontaneous remission. This is essentially an all-or-nothing approach. When those hopes go unmet, we are often plunged into the depths of despair. This makes it difficult for us to remain optimistic about trying other possible approaches.

When you have persistent pain, the key is not to wait for rescue. Each new moment offers the possibility of using the innate resources of your body to learn to regulate your pain and, ultimately, to resolve it. In the last chapter you learned about the power of being with your body and breathing. Your breath literally bridges what seems like a gap between mind and body and forges a partnership between them.

The next step in solving the puzzle of pain is to learn how to **FEEL in the same ways your body feels.** This means that instead of spacing out or dissociating from your body so that you don't feel as much, it's important to learn to tune in mindfully to your full array of body sensations, to recognize what your body is communicating to you. When you bring your mind, heart, and spirit to your body experience, then your full energy is available for healing.

No doubt you have become familiar with many of your pain patterns, the warning signals, the remedies that work the fastest and last the longest, and those that don't. During this chapter, we will start by using some fresh perspectives to map out your current pain terrain in such a way that you can begin to view the map as a locator of solutions as well as problems.

In her book *Turning Suffering Inside Out*, Darlene Cohen writes, "It takes not a little courage to watch ... your whole [pain] cycle. You go from a high-functioning person dealing effectively with chronic pain to increasing irritability as you get more tired and the pain gets worse. Finally you're facing all-out defeat and inrushing despair. At this point, you choose comfort even if that means depravity, and there's blessed spaciousness again before the pain starts anew. If you can watch this whole cycle—all without wincing, blinking, turning away, with your eyes open at every stage—you are a warrior."[1]

Map Your Pain Terrain:
Find Out How Bad Your Pain Really Is

So, aside from becoming a warrior because it seems like a pleasant fantasy, what can you hope to gain from focusing more directly on feeling your pain cycle? This is a key question when you have probably worked hard NOT to focus on the pain.

The greatest benefit is that focusing more effectively on your body and its sensations will give your brain the information it needs to turn on its natural regulation system effectively. For example, your knee or foot or hip or hand, wherever your pain center is, may hurt most of the time but not all of the time, or your pain levels may stay fairly constant but not bother you a certain percentage of your day. As you pay closer attention to your body sensations, you will begin to learn more about what seems to increase the pain and what relieves, diminishes, or changes your pain.

The question is, how can you focus on your pain *differently* than you do now in order to gain this kind of information? Part of the answer involves developing a different attitude toward the pain in your body, which the following exercises will help you to do.

If you have not done so recently, now is a good time to track your pain levels on an everyday basis for at least a week (although I recommend that you do so for at least a full month). Even if you have kept close track of daily pain fluctuations before, even as recently as when reading Chapter One, track them again, this time with the added dimension of tracking emotional pain and stress levels along with physical pain. Use a scale of 0–10, with zero representing no pain sensation and 10 representing severe pain. Monitoring your emotional pain simultaneously will give you additional information that will be very helpful. Suggested categories[2] are:

Physical Pain	Emotional Pain and Stress
0 No painful physical sensation	0 No negative emotional reaction
1–4 Low-intensity pain sensation	1–4 Minimal level of negative motion
5–6 Medium-intensity pain sensation	5–6 Moderate negative emotion
7–8 Significant pain, difficulty moving	7–8 Significant negative emotions
9–10 Severe pain with inability to move, minimal activity, bedridden	9–10 Severe depression, anxiety, despair; difficulty thinking

Exercise: Keep a Pain Notebook

I strongly recommend, if you haven't already done so, that you purchase a small pocket-size notebook that you use only as a pain diary. Choose three consistent times a day to rate your pain levels—for example, during your shower every morning, as you sit down to eat lunch, and just before bed. When you're ready to evaluate your pain, pay attention to the following:

First, give your physical pain a number from 0 to 10 and indicate your activity at the time (for example, watching TV, working at a computer, reading the paper, or cooking a meal). Then write down your emotional reaction to the physical pain and/or other life events and give them a number using the 0–10 scale above. Finally, at the end of the day, add up your three ratings of your physical pain and your three ratings of emotional reaction. Divide both by 3 to get your daily average and record this in your notebook.

Eventually you will begin to see pain patterns more clearly. Your pain diary can be used for multiple purposes: tracking your physical and emo-

tional pain levels, providing a place to record medications taken and results of self-treatment activities, keeping notes for meetings with various pain professionals to review your progress accurately, and noting all of the recommendations you receive. Before long, you will begin to see the value of keeping all this information in one location.

↶ SALLY, Part I

Sally had chronic pelvic pain resulting from complications related to a hysterectomy. Although she believed that she understood her pain well enough to know that it was constant and unrelenting in its severity, she agreed to keep a pain diary at my request. Since Sally used her computer for several hours every day while working, she decided to make pain graphs three times a day. For the first two weeks, she was surprised to discover that her pain was worst when she first woke up and again when she went to bed. Her daily physical pain average was 8, and her daily emotional pain average was a 7. She was also surprised that her emotional pain was so high. Sally commented, "I guess I'm more angry at the doctor who performed my hysterectomy than I thought I was. I really found out how bad I still feel about that whole experience and how angry I am that I have to deal with this chronic pain problem."

We were able to use several strategies to help Sally lower her pain levels while she was lying in bed before getting up and again at night before falling asleep. Once she was able to lower her first and last pain levels of the day reliably, Sally had more confidence that she could lower her pain levels at other times. Within a month, her pain average was 5. Once she learned to manage her negative thoughts about her doctor and her anxiety about how long her pain had lingered, her pain levels dropped to 4.

Sally told me later that the pain diaries had been very helpful:

"At first, I was angry with you for making me do them. Then I realized that they really were helping me learn what I needed to learn to get out of pain. Now I really don't want to stop doing them until I'm down to a one or two." And that was a process that took Sally about two more months.

Develop an Attitude of Openness, Curiosity, and Neutrality Toward *All* Body Sensations

Author Darlene Cohen, who has suffered from debilitating arthritis pain, tells the story of how she walked to the San Francisco Zen Center to eat lunch once a week as a treat. Sometimes she was in so much pain that she could not make it up the steps and would have to drag herself back home. She questioned herself, "What is it about walking that feels so tiring?" She then became aware that the most stressful, and therefore the most painful, aspect of walking was when she put the weight of her foot on the pavement. She realized that her joints got a rest when they were in the air. By *focusing on the foot in the air*, rather than the one on the pavement, Cohen was able to increase her stamina significantly and never again failed to climb the steps at the Zen Center.

a. *Try Cohen's exercise if you have any type of lower body pain. What are some variations that would work with pain in other parts of your body? How can you focus on body experience that has the least impact for you? Experiment until you have some success.*
b. *Focus on one of your pain patterns as if you were preparing a presentation for an academic class. How can you explain to others what is most hurtful about your pain?*

Exercise: Make Sense of Your Body's Sensations

Eugene Gendlin[3] was a pioneer in both the art and science of a method he called *Focusing*. Gendlin emphasizes the importance of discovering "the felt sense," which he describes as a *bodily* awareness related to a situation, person, or event rather than a mental awareness. The felt sense encompasses everything you feel and know about a given subject at a given time—encompasses it and communicates it to you all at once rather than detail by detail, or one part at a time. Developing your *felt sense* is another important technique related to the map of your pain terrain.

Peter Levine has made good use of Gendlin's focusing approach in Somatic Experiencing® (SE), his method of working with body experience related to trauma. Dr. Levine emphasizes that the felt sense is the medium through which we understand *all* sensation, and that it reflects our *total* experience at a given moment. Tuning into the felt sense keeps us from having to interpret what is happening based on information received from each separate part of the body.[4]

Peter Levine suggests a technique[5] that will help you to occupy your body more fully, and help to awaken your felt sense:

Take a gentle pulsing shower or bath for at least 10 minutes each day. Put your full awareness into the area where the water is pulsing. Let your awareness rotate to each part of the body as you rotate it under or in the water. Practice holding each part of your body under the water—face, hand, leg, foot, neck, upper back, middle and thoracic back, lower back, etc. Pay attention to each sensation whether numb, painful, or pleasant.

Use some variation of this exercise for several days or a week. What do you notice? What has shifted in your felt sense of your body after several water massages?

↶ SALLY, Part II

Sally learned about the felt sense by completing some of the exercises in this chapter. During one of the exercises, Sally made an important discovery. She realized that she did not know how her pain really *felt*. "I knew I felt bad but I didn't understand that the worst part is the burning sensations in my abdomen linked with the fear that I have when I feel the burning that it will only get worse and never stop."

Sally learned to stay with the sensations of burning and fear. As she did so for 5–10 minutes, the burning and fear became part of a stream of awareness that felt and seemed more neutral to her. Gradually she became aware of other sensations in her feet and arms and hands that engaged her curiosity and then began to feel more positive to her. After several sessions of working with the felt sense of her pelvic pain, Sally found that the most intense types of pain in her abdomen, the burning and stabbing sharp pain sensations, became softer and more tolerable.

Rebalance Your Daily Rhythms

Another aspect of learning about and turning on the body's natural pain regulation system is getting to know the daily rhythms in your everyday life. These rhythms might include times devoted to waking up, eating, exercise, rest, work, and play. Your daily routines can reveal accurate awareness of your natural biorhythms *or* they may expose conflicts about your body's natural rhythms and needs.

It is typical for people in pain to discover that their daily routines actually support *staying in pain* instead of *finding relief*. For example, one of my pain clients had to stop working because her job as a designer required her to stand on her feet all day. It was hard to give herself permission to rest, but that is what her body most needed

and responded to. She rearranged her schedule to include manda-
tory rest periods during both mornings and afternoons. These rest
periods included planned time for a nap each day, time for 15- to
30-minute mindfulness meditations, time to review audiotapes of
our sessions together, and time to sit in her garden. After a few weeks
of this slower rhythm, her pain levels were down by almost 50%.

Get Your Priorities Straight!

Even if you feel certain that your daily rhythms are ordered toward
wellness, sometimes a slight change can be the tipping point in your
self-care/pain equation. Any treatment plan for chronic pain will
include many different types of activities to help you shift from pain
to comfort or even pleasure.

Include one selection from each of the following treatment categories (first introduced to you in Chapter One) in your menu of
daily rhythms this week. Make necessary changes to incorporate this
more intensive focus for self-treatment for a few days or for an entire
week. Feel free to experiment beyond what is listed here. If you've
thought about a new method to try, this might be just the right time.

A chiropractor friend of mine[6] tells her pain patients: "Learn
something new. Take up painting, learn a new language, study music.
Get your neurons firing in a whole new way." This is good advice.
Here are some options to help you feel your way to a new direction:

1. **Body-focused therapy** (massage therapy, Alexander technique,
   Pilates, Somatic Experiencing,® Feldenkrais exercises, acupuncture, chiropractic care, exercise program, heat and cold therapy,
   electrical stimulation, biofeedback, etc.).
2. **Mind-Body-Heart-Spirit methods** (biofeedback, breathing techniques, imagery, hypnosis, meditation, yoga, cognitive-behavioral
   therapy, and energy psychology or energy medicine techniques).
3. **Pain-lowering diet and supplements.** Choose fresh (organic if

possible) fruit and vegetables, especially greens. Limit yourself to anti-inflammatory fats—oily fish and eggs with omega-3, flaxseed and flaxseed oil, pumpkin seeds, mackerel and herring, olive oil, salmon, sardines, and walnuts. Substitute whole grains for white bread and rice, and substitute complex carbohydrates that convert to proteins (beans, nuts) in the place of simple carbohydrates that convert rapidly to sugar (foods and drinks made with white flour, pasta, sugars). Include supplements and vitamins such as calcium and magnesium.

4. **Pain medications and medical treatment**[7] as needed. If you haven't recently reviewed your medications, please consider with your doctor your use of the following: steroidal anti-inflammatories; non-steroidal anti-inflammatories (NSAIDs) including Ibuprofen, Alleve, Mobic, Toradol; muscle relaxants; opioids such as Oxycontin and Vicodin; antidepressants such as Zoloft or Celexa; anticonvulsants including Neurontin or Tegretol. Start low and go slow until you reach the dose that gives you maximum relief with minimum side effects. Caution: *Never* make a change in your medication without consulting your prescribing physician.

Other medical interventions might include **nerve blocks** such as injections of lidocaine or an epidural block, which can be helpful for nerve pain. The results will vary from hours to days or weeks. There are no lasting results for anyone.[8]

Trigger point injections are analgesic injections into hypersensitive areas of tendons, muscles, or ligaments. These are especially useful for referred pain and muscle spasms. A similar effect can be obtained through cold sprays and stretching, or trigger point therapy.

Electrical and ultrasound stimulation including TENS (transcutaneous "through the skin" electrical nerve stimulation) is designed to stimulate nerves to turn on other sensations such as tingling that can mask pain signals and perhaps stimulate the body's natural pain relievers such as endorphins. Ultrasound can be particularly helpful with acute injury or reinjury.

5. **Sleep.** Don't forget sufficient sleep when you consider your priorities for your daily rhythms. (How many hours do you get? How many do you *need?*)

Optional: For support, partner (via phone or email) with someone who cares about you before you begin to change your daily rhythms. Review your existing daily routines in the above areas. Find out what your partner suggests that you add, subtract, or re-sequence in your daily rhythms. Create a self-treatment plan that brings the best results with the least amount of effort from you.[9] What rearrangement or changes in your priorities or daily rhythms seem to make sense in boosting pain relief for you? Where do you feel that your daily schedule is out of balance? If you need to find more energy so as not to feel overwhelmed by the various changes discussed in this chapter, ask your "buddy" for ideas about how to keep your mind open and your body willing to explore some of these possibilities.

Use Your Body's Good Sense

One of the advantages in learning how to regulate your pain rather than holding out for the magic bullet (i.e., zero pain levels all the time) is that self-regulation skills provide a way of making your pain more predictable *so that your **life** can become more predictable.* Self-regulation of pain also appears to facilitate steadiness or greater comfort across time, which promotes increased confidence and inner strength.

Because the felt sense is related to biological rhythms and cycles, it is actually possible to self-regulate your experience of pain simply by allowing your sensation cycles to ebb and flow naturally. By noticing and learning to trust your own natural rhythms, you relax and allow a sensation to unfold at its own pace. In this way you'll see that it will shift automatically into a different sensation, feeling, or awareness. Your body *is* resilient, with an astounding ability to heal itself. The good news here is that you don't have to push the river. Sometimes, in fact, it's pushing the river that causes the pain.

Exercise: Regulate Discomfort through Breathing and the Felt Sense

Sit with some discomfort in your body for a few minutes without trying to change it. As you breathe gently and easily, notice what happens naturally as time flows by. Then focus on a pleasurable area in your body. As you breathe gently and easily, notice what happens with this sensation as time flows by. Repeat this exercise with neutral sensation (sensation that is neither positive nor negative, such as an area of your face that is neither tight with tension nor pleasantly relaxed) and then repeat it again with a positive sensation. At any time you become distracted, take a break, and then refocus again, starting with your breath.

What do you notice about the progression of any pain sensation? Does it shift into other types of sensation and awareness?

⤳ SALLY, Part III

When Sally completed the exercise above, she discovered that the burning in her abdomen began to feel different as she stayed with her breathing and kept focusing her awareness on the pain sensations. At first they were almost unbearable—a 9 or 10 on her pain scale. Gradually, however, Sally noticed that the breathing helped her create a feeling of spaciousness in her abdomen. When she searched for a neutral sensation, she noticed that the bottoms of her feet were more comfortable and cool than her abdomen, a sense that increased as she kept her focus there.

Finally, she was able to find a positive sensation in her chest when her breathing seemed to bring a light, soothing feeling as her lungs expanded. Learning how focusing helped her connect with different types of sensation gave Sally more options in her experiential world and helped her to feel less trapped and hopeless.

Exercise: **Take Your Pain Apart**

A somewhat different method of tapping into your self-regulatory system is to focus on your pain in such a way that you begin to notice variations in it, and as you become more aware of those variations, the pain begins to lose its rigid totality. Dr. Jeffrey Zeig, an expert in the use of Ericksonian hypnosis, calls this "the Farrah Fawcett principle."[10]

The story goes that Dr. Zeig was working in a hospital setting years ago when, during lunchtime, several staff members were looking at a magazine photograph of actress Farrah Fawcett. Some members of the lunch group began to make negative comments about imperfections they observed in different parts of her body. By the time they had finished their analysis, Farrah Fawcett no longer appeared attractive to any of them!

You can practice this principle by working with the following exercise[11] to help change the rigid patterning of your pain:

Focus on the edges of your pain in your body. Ask yourself what the pain sensations look like or feel like. What do they remind you of? Where do you feel they are coming from? Can you imagine what is generating them? Sit quietly, open for any answer that may come from your creative mind. The answer may be in the form of another thought, sound, image, feeling, or picture. What comes up?

Next, imagine the qualities of the pain sensations themselves. What is their shape or size at this moment? Can you change the shape or size in any way? Can you shrink the pain area? Can you change its texture? Can you move the pain to another part of your body like your toe, a finger, or an earlobe where it will bother you less? What color do you associate with the sensations? Can you get the color to change in any way or perhaps to fade?

If the sensations remind you of an object, such as a knife, can you manipulate the object to regulate the pain? Can you remove the knife, for example, or put it back in its case? Does this make a difference in the pain you feel?

Finally, think about what makes you feel more comfortable when you have this kind of pain. What gives you the most reliable relief? Is it one of the five pain blockers you identified during Chapter One? Or is it something else that you think of right now . . . like a whirlpool bath . . . an afternoon lying in a hammock reading a novel . . . lying on the beach on a warm summer day . . . swimming or snorkeling in warm tropical water?

Can you imagine this relief going right to the center of your symptoms? To the core of what is causing the pain in this area?

Take a few moments to appreciate and acknowledge any changes that occur in your pain. Then gradually return your attention to this page. Read through the exercise again, this time noting what seemed to make a significant difference. How can you use this information in the future?

Goal for Chapter Two: After you've read quickly through this chapter for the first time, decide on one goal to focus on, such as discovering how the felt sense can help you reduce your pain levels by a half point. Then move through this material more slowly, practicing the techniques, completing some of the exercises and keeping your goal in mind. Remember, your goal must reflect where you truly want to put your energy even if this aim does not seem related to this chapter's focus on self-regulation. (Trust me, it probably is related in a way you might not imagine.) The most important part of setting a goal is to make it truly *yours*—not mine or what someone else believes you need to accomplish.

Write your pain goal in your pain notebook or on a bookmark for repeated reference and easy access.

SUMMARY: In this chapter you learned several different ways of focusing on the natural rhythms of the body's self-regulation system. We reviewed ways of developing curiosity and openness to body sensations. We learned a way to have a neutral observational focus on your pain areas. We explored how to awaken your body's "felt sense" through the flow of water over different parts of your body—and by just sitting with various body sensations for the purpose of noticing their natural ebb and flow.

You considered the importance of exploring your daily rhythms of pain and comfort, and of getting your priorities straight in terms of your personal daily treatment plan. You have taken your pain sensations apart to find out how this might shift your pain experience. The final exercise below combines your breathing techniques from Chapter One with the important skill of *pendulation,* which builds on the awareness of your felt sense.

Body Awareness Skill #2

FEEL: Breathe to Find Comfort as well as Pain

In this exercise, you will learn how to use the breath, your ability to focus on your body's sense (the felt sense), and the power of verbal self-suggestions to begin to regulate your discomfort.

"Pendulation"[12] refers to one of the most basic rhythmic patterns of our organism. Everything in our physical experience moves out and in, back and forth, beginning at the most primitive, foundational level with the breath cycle. This rhythm can be thought of as similar to the movements of a constantly swinging pendulum.

The principle of pendulum movement is that the movement on one side is identical to the movement on the other. Pendulum rhythm compensates and balances. The sympathetic branch of the nervous system turns on hyper-reactivity and freezing throughout the body when triggered by any signal of danger. This is related to the freeze/fight/flight response. The sympathetic cycle that stimulates these trauma reactions eventually turns on the parasympathetic restorative cycle, where there is relative calm. When there is persistent pain, this natural cycle has been interrupted. The practice of pendulation helps to revive the basic regulatory rhythms of the nervous system.

Set aside 20 minutes or so to complete this exercise. Make sure that phones are unplugged or turned off and that you have minimized intrusive distractions. As always, you are invited to modify the directions in any way that will be helpful to you.

1. *Begin by focusing on your breathing cycle as it is right now in the current moment. Complete a few breathing cycles of the breath method you chose in the first chapter—for example, calming breath, foursquare or circular breathing, purifying breath, or your own preferred method. Imagine the breath or healing light around you flowing into the areas of discomfort. Keep focusing on the breath as you focus on the safe place in your body that is a refuge from pain. Sit with any sensations that you notice and allow your awareness to follow their natural ebb and flow in and through your body.*

2. *After a short break if you need one, return to your focus on the breath and body sensations. The pendulum rhythm offers a highly effective way to regulate pain.*

   a. *Explore the edges of this pain center as if you were constructing a map of it, or as if you were pulling up a chair and sitting next to it, noticing all that you can about this body area. Now focus on the place in your body that feels the farthest away, or most different from that discomfort. Explore the edges of this area, again imagining that you are creating an internal map of this area of relative comfort.*

a. *With the mental focus of a neutral observer, bridge back and forth with your awareness of the felt sense from the area of relative comfort to the pain and back again. Do this bridging cycle several times.*

For example, first notice the area of discomfort and study it objectively as if for a scientific presentation. Then notice the area you identified that feels far away and very different from that. What do you notice as you bridge back and forth? What happens if you reverse the order (discomfort first and then the more comfortable area)? You may find that you begin to sense a third type of sensation that is different from the first two.

c. *Next, add the breath to your bridging. Experiment with focusing on the felt sense of comfort as you breathe in and the area of discomfort as you breathe out. (Reverse this order if that feels better.) This process might go something like the following: breathe in— notice the tightness and soreness; breathe out—notice the feeling of comfort in your feet. Repeat this pendulation cycle using the breath at least 5 times. What do you notice in terms of the rhythms of your felt sense? Did you become aware of something like a third state in your body?*

d. *Finally, add cue words or self-suggestions to deepen the different state you have been creating while pendulating back and forth. Experiment with words on the "in" breath such as "release" or "relax" or "calm" and others on the out breath such as "now" or "deeply" or "letting go." Continue until you find a matched pair that seems to anchor a positive response in your nervous system. You are using the hypnotic principle of ideodynamic healing[13] to make a powerful impact on the dynamic processes of the body by having the mind focus on important key words. Your breath and your mental focus have become an important bridge between mind and body.*

In the next chapter, we add the element of relaxation to what you have learned so far about using the breath and your body's sense to further awaken natural healing cycles. As you reflect on what you've learned during this chapter, have you been able to further decrease your pain? What would it take to shift your pain another half or full point lower on the scale? If you feel you need more practice of the skills presented in this chapter, consider doing a mini-review first before moving on to Chapter Three.

CHAPTER THREE

Relax
Feel the Pleasure Around Pain

Why is relaxation such an important part of pain treatment? The short answer is that if your body is enjoying pleasant relaxation, you will be less likely to experience discomfort or pain. This is because relaxation techniques seem to help reconnect your body with remembered states of letting go of tension, stress, and pain.

Research shows that relaxation has many benefits. Among other effects, relaxation can decrease metabolism, blood pressure, heart rate, breathing rate, and muscle tension while increasing slower brain waves.[1] For just about anyone who is struggling with a pain condition, it is important to master simple relaxation practices that are reliably soothing and calming to counteract the effects of everyday anxiety that tend to push pain levels higher. There is also some evidence that individuals who regularly practice the relaxation response are less reactive to various stress hormones, even at times when they are not practicing.[2]

When you are in pain or anxious about whether you will be, your muscles are tense, whether you are aware of the tension or not. Tense muscles require more oxygen than relaxed ones, yet the blood vessels that carry oxygenated blood unfortunately are often constricted by surrounding muscle tissue, which prevents these supplies from reaching the parts of the muscles that need them most. Poor oxygenation of tense muscles then tends to result in greater discomfort and stiffness. General fatigue also occurs because keeping muscles tense drains much more energy than keeping muscles relaxed.

Ongoing states of muscle tension tend to be related to the fight/flight/freeze response that is part of your body's reaction to overwhelming stress and the activation of the sympathetic nervous system in response to real or imagined threat. If sympathetic activation is prolonged, related chemicals of adrenaline and cortisol maintain tension in the muscles, and this creates further exhaustion and pain. Over time, muscle tension can become habitual, sending signals to the brain that fear of threat is still present, which pulls your body even further away from relaxation.[3]

When pain and physical tension become chronic, you may reach a point where you are no longer even aware how constricted your muscles have become, and releasing or relaxing them becomes almost impossible. In fact, if you try to relax, your muscles may tighten even more because they have forgotten what letting go and relaxation feel like.

If you have been in pain for a long time, be prepared to feel off-balance when learning relaxation. Starting to let go of tension might feel a little frightening, as if you are losing control of your body. If this is the case for you, relaxation needs to be relearned. As you practice the relaxation techniques in this chapter, remember that you *are* in control even if you don't feel that you are. You can stop when you wish, start when you wish, or even tense up again if you need to.

It is crucial, however, that you learn to release tension, because only when your body finds relaxation can you reverse the damaging biochemical processes caused by stress. Bringing about the positive hormonal changes related to relaxation will dramatically reduce your pain levels. Eventually, when you become skilled at relaxing your mind-body system, you will be able to recognize when muscle tension is building up and will automatically be able to shut it off.

One physical relaxation technique that relieves many kinds of pain involves actually creating *more* tension in your body first, and then releasing it very gradually. This method, called the "tension-release" or progressive relaxation technique, helps you learn to **regulate** the sensations of relaxation—much like in the last chapter, when you learned to begin to regulate sensations of pain. We will practice the tension-release technique at the end of this chapter.

Correct Your Limiting Beliefs about Body Relaxation

Although you may agree in theory that relaxation is important, you may not have a reliable method that works well for you. And, you may even have had some negative experiences that led to the formation of beliefs that now block your ability to create relaxation in your body. Before you begin relaxation training, we will examine and correct some common limiting beliefs to prevent them from blocking your practice.

Please take a few moments to reflect on each of these beliefs about relaxation as it relates specifically to you. This section is designed to remove negative beliefs related to past relaxation experiences so that the tools you work with in this chapter will be more effective. As you read these sections, notice any reactions in your body. Pay particular attention to any strong "positive" or "negative" feedback from your body, as this will help you learn more about your body's natural feedback system.

1. I have tried many ways to relax and they just don't work to reduce my pain. Perhaps past approaches you have tried were too complex. One of the simplest ways to approach relaxation is by learning about the relaxation reaction that is already hard-wired into the human organism. There are numerous ways to activate what Dr. Herb Benson, professor at Harvard, has called *the relaxation response*.

As a cardiologist, Dr. Benson conducted research on the effects of biofeedback and meditation on stress-related health issues such as high and low blood pressure. Benson discovered that for any disorder caused or worsened by stress, methods that stimulate the relaxation response are helpful. He coined the term "relaxation response" to refer to the body's method of regulating its own physiological systems through a series of changes in metabolism, breath rate, heart rate, alpha waves, blood pressure, and muscle tension.[4]

As Benson explored the effects of different relaxation approaches, he discovered that each one stimulated a set of slightly different physiological changes. For example, transcendental meditation, yoga, and hypnotic suggestion all decreased oxygen consumption, respiration, heart rate, and blood pressure, and increased alpha waves in the brain. Progressive body relaxation techniques, where you gradually tense and then relax all of the major muscle groups in the body, do not necessarily promote these changes, but they do decrease muscle tension, which is not as true of the other approaches.

People in pain need to find a path to relaxation that works best for them. Much as pain is a very individual experience, so is relaxation. Benson's research has suggested that the relaxation response can be created just as successfully during active exercise (such as bicycle riding) as it can through more passive methods (such as listening to music or a relaxation tape). This effect has been duplicated using a type of hypnotic suggestion called "active alert" hypnosis,[5] which dispels the myth that hypnosis or relaxation can only happen when you are quiet with your eyes closed. For some people, swimming or other rhythmic exercise provides the best method of relaxation. For others, golfing or other active sports such as tennis or soccer seem to unlock the relaxation response.

What is required is the courage and patience to keep exploring until you find the right combination that tips you away from pain, tension, depression, and despair and toward vitality, peace, comfort, and well-being. Regardless of the method used, creating the relaxation response in your body can only happen with regular practice. Yet if you find yourself resisting the "work" of practicing relaxation, remember that even if you merely think about relaxation, you will get some of the same benefits as if you had practiced the exercises exactly as they are written.

2. I have trouble relaxing my body so I guess I'm just going to be stuck with this pain. This belief implies that achieving relaxation in the body is an absolute must for resolving chronic pain. However, one of the most common techniques, muscle relaxation, may not help significantly or may provide only temporary relief for pain conditions unless they are caused by physical tension. For example, nerve pain does not usually respond well to muscle relaxation.

Yet for certain types of pain and for certain individuals, physical relaxation can be highly useful. For example, research has shown that relaxation techniques are particularly effective with headache pain. Several studies have found that relaxation training used as the only treatment produced a 38% improvement for people with migraine headaches and a 45–70% improvement for those with tension headaches.[6]

Even if your pain is not tension-based, *anxiety* almost always is a component of the chronic pain equation. Suggestions and methods for body relaxation are one of the *most proven* treatments for reducing or eliminating virtually all types of anxiety. High levels of anxiety and stress tend to decrease the threshold for pain so that a more anxious person becomes more sensitive to initial pain sensations (especially increases in pain) and may also perceive pain sensations as being worse than someone who tends not to worry. So even if you don't use relaxation techniques to reduce your pain sensations directly, they will be helpful in reducing the anxiety, stress, and worry that drive your pain levels up and cause you to spiral downward.

When pain cycles begin, the worrier tends to worry about how bad the pain will get, and these kinds of anxious thoughts can actually intensify the perceptions of pain. Thus, anxiety can contribute to a vicious circle of pain—anxiety about the pain, followed by more pain, then more anxiety about the pain, and so on. The relaxation response may help people who worry to tolerate pain more easily and therefore actually decrease the intensity of their pain. Because anxiety can intensify pain and pain often intensifies anxiety, this is the one of the most important patterns to learn to reverse.

3. I relax too much now as it is. I have already had to decrease my activity level so much that if I spend more time relaxing, I'm afraid I will never recover from pain. The fears behind this statement are all too real. Sometimes it's true that our loved ones have become impatient with our progress and resent having to take over more chores because we must do less. The thought of planning more time to relax in these circumstances seems out of the question and, we fear, may increase the stress in an already strained relationship.

If relationship issues are at the heart of your concerns about relaxing more, now is probably a very good time to have an honest talk with your spouse, partner, friend, or family member. It's important that both of you are honest about your feelings and needs. It is natural for a loved one who must "pick up the slack for you" over a long interval of time to feel resentful about the time you can devote to meditation and rest. (It may be a "hard sell" to loved ones that your most important work right now is to learn to relax your mind and body.) You may need to acknowledge the valid reasons for any resentment between the two of you and to explore ways of rebalancing the work of the relationship.

For example, if your partner is doing the work of shopping and making meals, you may agree to plan menus, order groceries online, and clean up. If you are unable to contribute to cleaning the house, perhaps you can take over paying the bills, returning phone calls, or conducting written correspondence for both of you. Such an approach is aimed at helping you contribute more equal time when you are unable to contribute equal energy or money.

There is one other important issue related to this belief. There is a huge difference between spending big blocks of time in inactivity and experiencing *enjoyable* relaxation. How much time do you actually spend during your day where the only goal is relaxation? Take a few minutes to compute that total for at least one full day. What is your guesstimate?

If you spend more than 2–3 hours experiencing completely enjoyable relaxation during your day on a regular basis, then I would agree that it's time to increase your activity level. I suspect what's true, however, is that you spend much more time than that struggling with questions related to this issue: "Is it really OK for me to take a nap when I slept for 10 hours last night?" or "How can I say no to the movies when I say no too much as it is?"

Sometimes this kind of intense self-questioning and struggling can stem from longstanding internal conflicts among parts of the self. It's important to understand that if you wrestle with these kinds of conflicts, it may not feel enjoyable, especially at first, to concentrate and focus your attention in unfamiliar ways. We will examine this topic later on during Chapters Six and Eight and offer help for this kind of barrier.

4. When my body is in intense pain, I simply cannot relax, no matter what I do. From a strictly physiological perspective, this statement may be true. A body in pain may not be able to relax due to the chemical changes that accompany intense and/or prolonged pain. In these circumstances, we are in a state of fight/flight/ freeze emergency response, which turns on powerful chemical and electrical changes in the nervous system. These chemical changes contribute to increased muscle tension, heart rate, blood pressure, respiratory rate, and an increased flow of stress hormones such as adrenaline and cortisol. The chemistry of the fight/flight/freeze response is in dramatic opposition to the chemicals that accompany the relaxation response. Therefore, your body may indeed be initially quite resistant to relaxation when you are in a state of intense pain and alarm.

If you understand this chemical process, however, you can begin to intervene in states of activated fight/flight/freeze response more and more effectively. It is recommended that you first develop confidence in the method of relaxation training you have selected by using it at times when your pain is at lower levels. The main point here is to **intervene as early as possible** in your pain cycle, as Eric learned to do.

⌐ ERIC

Eric, one of my clients who had more than twenty knee surgeries, learned that he needed to track his pain very carefully. When it increased to 4 or 5 on a 10-point scale, he would intervene as soon as possible by lying down and listening to a prepared relaxation tape or by using his portable biofeedback machine while icing his knee. At first, it took him almost an hour to achieve enough relaxation for the pain to decrease. And the relaxation response would dissipate fairly quickly when he started moving around again. It was a struggle for him to spend even more time than usual trying to relax and having such insignificant results.

A year later, however, he can sit down and rest for 10–15 minutes by quieting his mind and icing his knee. His pain levels rarely rise above 3, and if they do, he is confident that he can reduce them again relatively quickly so that he can resume regular activity.

Exercise: Intervene Early in Your Pain Cycle to Achieve Reliable Relaxation

For the next day or so, practice creating the relaxation response sooner than you normally would intervene in your pain cycle when your pain levels are *relatively* low. Your goal is to use the relaxation response to keep your pain in a range that is about one point lower than the average range of your pain now.

For example, if your pain currently averages 8–10 points on a 10-point scale, you would attempt to use relaxation training when the pain is around 6–8 (rather than when it is 8–10) so that you can lower your overall pain range to 5–7. This might mean that you are doing relaxation training early in the morning and/or that you use it more frequently during the day. Challenge yourself to commit to this plan for at least one day. Use one or more of the following methods.

a. Try some variation of Benson's technique,[7] *which is the Relaxation Response we have been discussing above.*

Exercise: Steps to Achieve the Relaxation Response

1. Sit quietly in a comfortable position. If it helps to close your eyes, do so.

2. Progressively relax your muscles, starting with your feet and legs and moving up to the top of your head. If it helps, you can suggest to yourself, "Now I want to relax my feet," . . . etc. If this feels awkward, try starting with the top of your head and move down to your feet.

3. Breathe in through your nose with mouth closed. As you breathe out through your nose or mouth, think the words "let go." Be aware of any feeling of release. Continue for about 20 minutes. Breathe in . . . out . . . **let go;** *breathe in . . . out . . .* **let go.** *You can open your eyes to check the time, but do not set an alarm.*

4. *Maintain a permissive attitude and let relaxation take place at its own pace. Expect distracting thoughts; when these occur, ignore them by thinking, "Oh well," and then return to breathing—in . . . out . . .* **let go.**

5. *Practice once or twice daily but not within two hours following a meal. Practice at a time of day that brings the best results for you. (NOTE: Many people find that it's harder to concentrate immediately after a meal.)*

---

b. If you already have a relaxation tool that has helped before, such as an audiotape or guided meditation CD, dust it off and use it again. Make sure that the focus of whatever method you choose is on your awareness of your **body's** *experience of relaxation. (It's also possible to use a tool that, although it is not designed for body relaxation, consistently has that effect for you, as is true of many types of meditation and more active exercise methods.)*

c. Do an online search or interview other people with chronic or persistent pain about what works for them, and use this opportunity to try something that has stood the test of time for someone else.

5. Body relaxation does not work for *my* **kind of pain because it's nerve pain.** There actually is some evidence that body relaxation does not work as well for some types of pain as it does for others. Nerve pain is the least responsive to physical relaxation techniques.[8] Examples of nerve pain include peripheral neuropathy in the hands and feet, neuralgia and shingles, and carpal tunnel syndrome, in addition to "pinched" or "entrapped nerve" syndromes in the neck, joints, disc, and sciatic areas.

It is important to understand that *all* people with chronic pain have some degree of nerve pain. When nerves are traumatized or over-stimulated for a long period of time, they are not as accurate at distinguishing between pain and other types of sensations. They emit erroneous pain messages, keeping the nerves *hypersensitized*. The longer you are in persistent or chronic pain, the more sensitized your nerves may become, so that they literally become unable to recognize non-pain sensations. When this happens, persistent or chronic pain can create a vicious loop in the nervous system that causes pain to feel unrelenting. Because all sensation feels like the same pain, the nervous system magnifies even the smallest pain.

A dramatic example of this is phantom limb pain, when even after amputation, pain in the severed limb area persists in the absence of pain stimuli due to continued firing of nerve fibers in the dorsal horn pain gate area at the back of the spinal cord. Some experts (including pain pioneers Rod Melzack and Patrick Wall) believe that this "over-firing" pattern can become imprinted in the nervous system, becoming a problem in itself.

But even though nerve pain may be less responsive to body relaxation methods, this does not mean that you should not try them. Nerve pain will usually respond best to relaxation techniques that involve some type of gentle body movement or distraction, rather than mental and physical quieting. An example is the TENS unit, a pocket-sized, portable, battery-operated machine that sends electrical impulses to certain parts of the body to block pain signals and has a strong record with nerve pain. You might also explore activities such as creating artwork or listening to your favorite music. These hobbies are effective because they stimulate the relaxation response through the positive focus of an active mind while distracting the nervous system from its usual reactions.

Keep Relaxation Simple

Relaxation techniques sometimes do not work because they are too complex. One way of guaranteeing success with any task is to break it down into small, manageable steps. This is sometimes called *chunk-*

ing. For example, if you are struggling with a breathing exercise, challenge yourself to do the very smallest part you can do.

If you become too distracted by the thoughts that intrude into your concentration on the breath cycle, for example, keep it simple by focusing on the smallest part of the exercise such as breathing in, and let go of the rest of the exercise. If that step feels good and you are using Benson's method, maybe the next step is to add the word "breathe" (or another word that fits for you) while breathing in.

Another possibility is to take short, shallow breaths if that is easier at first rather than slow, deep ones. One of my clients told herself that the first few minutes when she practiced breathing and relaxation techniques might feel "weird" to her, but that her reaction would change if she stayed with it. So sometimes a "hang in there" reminder may help you be successful.

This process is a something like playing the childhood game of "pick up sticks" or the Jenga wooden block tower game. Your challenge is to begin with only one tiny step as a foundation. Then you must add another small step without disturbing the first one, and so on. If you take baby steps, you will find that you can move through *any* practice exercise more easily.

Another way to keep it simple is to find your "tipping point" for relaxation. If you play close (yet neutral) attention whenever you practice any form of relaxation, you will find the moment where all-encompassing pain begins to shift even a tiny bit. Then the challenge is to make further choices that continue the shift away from the "dark side" of pain in more little steps. This approach may be thought of as **chaining** or **stacking.** The idea is that if you link together several very small changes to create a chain, that chain will be more resistant to being broken than any one individual link. AND, most importantly, positive changes that are created in small incremental steps are much more likely to be integrated as *permanent* than sudden, dramatic ones, which tend to disrupt the equilibrium of the nervous system and ultimately be rejected.

Create Relaxation That You Actually Enjoy

People who experience chronic pain are notoriously out of practice at finding pleasure in their lives. Yet searching for moments of pleasure is one way of breaking through the chronic freezing or gridlock of the nervous system and interrupting hypersensitive nerve pain cycles.

Where can you start to look for pleasure? You might want to start with your senses other than those related to pain. For example, you might notice the pleasure of seeing, or more tactile or sensate pleasures of the body. Visit a museum, allow your eyes to feast on beautiful flowers or photographs, or create a beautiful light show with inexpensive prisms. You can also enjoy the pleasure of hearing beautiful music, Tibetan bells or wind chimes, or the sound of a waterfall or small fountain. And let's not forget the scent of a favorite flower, or your favorite food baking, of freshly cut grass, or a French soap.

People with impairment in one sense learn how to compensate by strengthening others. What would it be like to really view chronic pain as a sensate impairment and intentionally strengthen and broaden your abilities to experience pleasure through different sensory modalities?

And what about the positive effects of simple laughter and play? There is actually a large amount of research on the benefits of laughter for the body.[9] These include dramatic shifts in our internal chemistry such as reductions in stress hormones, increases in the number of killer cells available to fight disease and infection, and the release of endorphins, those hormones that make us feel good. The old cliché that "laughter is the best medicine" really is true.

You have probably heard of Norman Cousins, who treated his

cancer by watching funny movies for several hours each day. Cousins reported that his pain tolerance increased significantly after laughing for 10 minutes. If he laughed throughout the morning, he found that the rest of his day would be virtually pain-free.

Here are some suggestions to help you cultivate laughter daily in your life.[10]

1. *Make sure you never miss your favorite, reliably fun TV show. Include reruns, no matter how often you've seen them.*
2. *Be sure to read email jokes that come from your funniest friends.*
3. *Check out funny websites and bookmark them. These might include "pretty good jokes" on the Prairie Home Companion's website at www.phc.mpr.org, selections from www.jokesgalore.com, or www.cartoonbank.com.*
4. *Rent movie comedies, the sillier the better. Browse at your local video store or use Netflix. If you still want some ideas, research the American Film Critics' recommendations or other similar list of the top 100 funniest movies ever made.*

Develop a Relaxation Practice That Restores Body, Mind, Heart, and Spirit

If it is difficult to find relaxation in your body, sometimes it works to find other types of relaxation first. For example, you may need to find a method to quiet the chatter of your conscious mind that repeats negative messages like "This won't work" or "This doesn't matter."

Chronic pain is a disorder of the mind as well as the body, and of the heart as well as the spirit. Pain messages light up the center of emotions in the limbic system at the same time they are routed to other parts of the brain. When a pain signal is received, the limbic system sends a powerful group of emotional signals, including anger, panic, fear, or sadness. The limbic system also turns on hormones that affect your physical state and triggers changes in the brain's cortex that influence your thinking. And many experts view suffering that arises from pain as a spiritual issue. Chronic physical pain can be a way of understanding the deeper pain of the soul.

When you make time to focus on a relaxation practice, make sure to include "medicine for the mind." This may be a positive suggestion, such as "I can enjoy this focus on breathing and my body," or you may want to start with music or soothing sounds or even white background noise that can give your mind a place to rest.

Herb Benson suggests repeating words that are innately relaxing such as "one," "ocean waves," "love," or "peace." He has also conducted informal research in his clinical practice with assignments that his patients repeat words of faith that are important for them, with significant healing results.[11]

Time for spiritual meditation, chanting, and prayer can be an invaluable bridge to body relaxation. Finding sources of inspiration in the written word, in a spiritual community, or in the natural world of creation might be a good foundational step to build on. And for many people, there is no substitute for an active prayer life.

Recognize Your Body's "Yes" and "No" Responses to Relaxation

Sudden pain increases can let you know that you have pushed past safe physical, mental, or emotional limits and that you may need to *do nothing* until your body's feedback changes again. This may be your body's "no" response to your efforts to "try to" relax. If this seems to be true, learn to cultivate the art of doing nothing.

Years ago, I was in graduate school at Penn State and under huge pressure to finish my master's thesis along with multiple other projects by a firm deadline to complete my degree. Once I got to a certain level of exhaustion and worry during those last few weeks, I could no longer focus in any kind of productive way on my work.

Sometimes I could exercise or use some of the other steps in this chapter for relief, but if that time of "hitting the wall" came late at night, or at some other inconvenient time, I found that my body seemed to resist any and all attempts to let go of stress. At those times, I found that staring at my digital clock with large numbers was oddly restful. Basically, I learned to *vacate* my mind as well as my body until I felt an inner sense of balance and calm that I recognized as my body's "yes" response. This "yes" meant that I could then move on to other possibilities, such as listening to music or meditating, which would be successful in restoring mind, body, heart, and spirit.

The challenge here is to trust that your body's feedback *will* change. It always does—you read your body's different signals when you know you are ready to have a good sleep, a good cry, or a good laugh. Yet our fear is that any negative body feedback we receive will be never-ending.

For a simple experiment, practice reading each of the headings in this chapter (or a previous one). Tune into the reactions your body has toward each one. If you aren't sure, repeat or read further. Find the section in this chapter that seems to activate the most neutral or positive response, as well as the part that elicits the most resistance or negative reaction. What happens in your body that you label neutral or positive? What happens in your body that you label negative?

Eventually you can learn to read your body's feedback as its "yes" or "no" response and use these signals to make wise decisions about your needs. For now, if you'd like to take this further, practice reading the section that evokes the strongest negative response from your body. Then read the section that evokes the most positive or neutral response (or the least negative reaction) in your body. What happens? If you'd like, record your findings in your pain notebook (or make some mental notes).

Exercise: **Practice Pendulation to Counter the Fight/Flight/Freeze Response**

In the last chapter, we learned about the skill of pendulation. If you feel you need more practice with pendulation, this might be a good time for the following exercise (providing your body gives you its "yes" biofeedback). Pendulation is especially effective in allowing the body to relax and let go of tension and stress related to the fight, flight, and freeze response.

Unlike animals in the wild, the "civilized" human organism does not tend to go through the instinctual discharge of the freeze response, which leaves us vulnerable to constriction and pain. Nor can we run away or fight back against danger in most situations, and we are not encouraged to release shock and freezing responses when they occur. Deer freeze in the glare of headlights, and then tremble violently when the danger signaled by headlights is past. This trembling literally allows them to "shake off" the freeze response. After this discharge, they are able to run or move without any lasting impairment. Trauma experts believe that interruption of the freeze response (which wild animals rarely experience) contributes to *kindling* in humans, a process of over-firing in the nervous system that triggers symptoms of post-traumatic stress disorder as well as chronic pain and other health problems.

"Kindling"[12] is a complex process that has been compared to spontaneous combustion, a chemical chain reaction that occurs when materials reach a certain temperature. The term is used to explain how over-firing or neural excitability in the nervous system becomes self-perpetuating without additional external triggering. That can be why, even though what caused your pain is long past, the pain continues on and on.

Pendulation is one effective method that can begin to unlock the freezing and hypersensitive responses of the nervous system. The rhythm of pendulation is similar to breathing rhythms and other primitive biorhythms of the organism. Pendulation helps to activate basic regulatory rhythms and stops nervous system rigidity and random responses, thus interrupting all kinds of traumatizing pain, including nerve pain.

a. *First focus on an area where there is the least discomfort at this moment. You might want to start with the type of breathing cycle that works best for you (calming breath, etc.). Explore the edges of this place in your body. If it helps, move that area of the body (if possible) to learn more about the felt sense there (or put your hand gently on that body area).*

b. *Then focus on a place in your body that is on the periphery of the pain area (not at the center of it). Explore this area as if you were drawing a map or completing the drawing of your body.*

c. *With your thinking mind, first notice the calmer place and then notice the uncomfortable place. Bridge back and forth, back and forth, a few times.*

d. *Then add conscious breathing to the pendulation process. As you breathe in, focus on one area, and as you breathe out, focus on the other area. Complete this cycle several times until you notice that you are starting to feel something different in your body. Be curious about this new response and repeat the exercise if that feels useful.*

SUMMARY: This chapter gave you an opportunity to explore and correct limiting beliefs about body relaxation. You learned that the *relaxation response* is a natural response that can be turned on in many ways, including the use of sensory modalities other than body feeling. You've learned how the fight/flight/freeze response can create gridlock in the nervous system and lead to hypersensitivity of nerve cells. You then reviewed several ways to help create effective relaxation. Now we will practice the tension-release method as another approach to turn on the relaxation response.

Body Awareness Skill #3

RELAX Your Muscles, Relax Your Brain, Turn Off Pain

This exercise is built around the tension-release method to promote physical relaxation. NOTE: Discontinue this exercise if it increases your pain. If your pain is primarily nerve pain, you may want to skip this exercise and spend the time refining your skill with pendulation.

1. *Begin as usual by focusing on your breathing cycle as it is right now in the current moment. Complete a few breathing cycles of the breath method you chose in Chapter One—e.g. calming breath, foursquare or circular breathing, or purifying breath. Imagine the breath or the light around you flowing into the areas of discomfort. Keep focusing on the breath as you focus on the safe place in your body that feels like a* **refuge** *from pain. Sit with any sensations that you notice and allow your awareness to follow their natural ebb and flow in and through your body. Add key words while breathing in and out if this is helpful.*
2. *Begin to tighten progressively the muscle areas throughout your body as suggested in the next paragraph. If you are concerned that this will increase your pain further, or you receive feedback from your body that indicates a "no" response, move on to options 3 or 4 below.*

   Begin with your feet and legs and move up the body. When ready, tense the muscles in one foot and hold the tension as you hold your breath. Then release all the tension in your body as you release your breath by breathing out. Repeat this several times and then move to four or five other sites in the body (or right-left pairs of sites) and notice what effect you are getting. Usually by the third breath cycle there is a cumulative change of release or loosening. Notice how this affects your pain over the span of a day or two.

3. *A variation of this approach (if you want one) involves clenching your fist.*[13] *Take a moment and imagine that all your pain can flow into one or both hands. As you are aware of this transfer, clench your fist(s) as tightly as possible. Continue clenching (unless this causes more pain) until you can get a sense that the pain from different areas in your body is collecting there. Hold the fist(s) as tightly as possible along with your breath, and when you are ready, let go of your breath along with the muscles of your fist(s) very very slowly. Notice what kind of feeling this creates for you.*

4. *A VERY brief variation (only if you want one) is the marble technique.*[14] *Imagine that you are squeezing a marble in one of your hands—or actually do so with a marble, stone, or shell. The harder you squeeze the object you have chosen, the more comfortable you will feel. This is because as you squeeze the marble, you concentrate more of your body stress and tension into your hand. Let it go into the marble, which is very strong and can absorb an unlimited amount of discomfort. How does this feel? You can use your marble to deal with stress or increased pain at any time. Even if you don't have your marble with you, you can imagine holding it in your hand and you will get some of the same good feelings.*

CHAPTER FOUR

Imagine
Recreate Your Reality
of Living with Pain

Imagery is one of the best ways we have of tapping into the power of the creative imagination. Researchers have demonstrated that various types of imagery have a significant positive impact on physiological processes. Imagery has been found to lower blood pressure and heart rate, to decrease anxiety and depression, to reduce cholesterol and lipids, to speed healing from cuts, fractures, and burns, to enhance autoimmune function, and to reduce pain from arthritis and fibromyalgia, just to name a few of the successful applications.[1]

I have found that another major benefit of imagery is that because it can help improve mood and reduce pain, it is often useful in helping people withdraw from medications that are addictive or have created a physical or emotional dependence.

As with all the other chapters, read over the material here first, then use your sense of your body's "yes" and "no" responses to determine which skills or exercises are right for you now. Remember to set a goal or positive intention to guide your reading and practice, particularly in those areas that you feel drawn toward.

Imagery Taps the Eight Senses

Most of us believe that we have five senses to take in information about our physical world: vision, hearing, touch, taste, and smell.

There is fairly broad agreement about a sixth sense, the power of intuition.[2] Intuition refers to an instinctive belief or hunch without "objective" or "scientific" evidence about some aspect of our experience.

What are the other two senses I'm proposing? Both are expansions of the sense of touch. One is the *felt sense*, already introduced to you in Chapter Two, which is considered to be your *body awareness* or *body presence*. Becoming aware of your felt sense heightens your ability to heal whatever kind of pain you experience. Coupled with your intuition, you will be better able to sense what is best for your body at any particular stage of healing.

The eighth sense I am referring to is your **proprioceptive** sense.[3] This sense emerges from *proprioceptors*, which are nerve endings in your muscles, tendons, and joints that provide a sense of your body's position in space. Your proprioceptors record responses to a wide range of factors that stimulate a physical reaction, including heat, cold, electrical impulses, and drugs.

The proprioceptive sense allows you to be in greater attunement with different locations in your body and to make discriminations among them. By developing this sense, not only can you get an overall sense of body presence, you can also tune in to specific areas of your body that require special attention from you, or ones that offer resources for healing.

Through the rest of this chapter, we will consider how these eight senses are captured and expressed in different forms of imagery, which provide useful tools for working with body presence.

Turn On Your Brain's Creative Reality

You are probably already familiar with guided imagery. In my previous book, *Finding the Energy to Heal*, I reviewed several types of guided imagery that have been particularly useful in my clinical practice.[4] *Guided or structured imagery* can be considered a form of directed fantasy or daydreaming. When we use structured imagery, we guide our thought processes to invoke and use all of the senses. This type of imagery is effective primarily because it can sidestep limited thinking, logical and illogical assumptions, and psychological barriers such as fear and resistance.

A guided imagery approach sends healing messages encoded in the language of sensory suggestions and symbols into the right hemisphere of the brain, where they affect many primary functions. Some experts believe that in some cases imagery can even intervene at the cellular level, where it acts directly on the DNA.[5]

The second basic type of imagery emerges spontaneously in dreams or as a free association when given a more unstructured suggestion such as "Just see what comes to mind when you think about the pain in your back right now." This is a more passive, receptive use of imagery. Although it also has its place in the self-treatment of pain, we will not focus on this kind of imagery in this chapter. Perhaps you can "watch" for this type of imagery if it appears spontaneously after you have completed an exercise, or when you are falling asleep at night or just waking up in the morning. These are spontaneous gifts of the imagination and they, too, can be valuable healing resources.

How to Use Structured or Guided Imagery: There are several aspects of using structured or guided imagery for pain, discussed point by point below.

1. First, it's important to develop the ability to perceive and express any event or experience as a sensory image. It is usually best to start with your strongest modality. We can begin with a felt-sense image, visual image, auditory image, kinesthetic or tactile image, a postural or body movement proprioceptive image, or even a taste or smell image.

2. Next, we connect *all* our remaining senses with the image and amplify our connection with the image so that it is as full as possible.
3. We then test the strength of the image to make sure that it is stronger than the pain or targeted problem we are working with.
4. Finally, we practice using the image to meet the desired goal.

Guided or structured imagery is always **interactive.** That is, there is an interplay between the instructions suggested by a guided exercise and *you*, the person forming the images. In most cases, how you respond to each suggestion you are given will influence the next set of instructions, and so on.

⌐ MARIA

I asked Maria, a thirty-year-old woman suffering from whiplash caused by a recent car accident, to imagine and describe the area of greatest pain. She described the center of her pain as a silver sphere about 4 inches in diameter on her left cervical spine. When I suggested that Maria become fully connected to this image using all of her senses, she reported that she could hear a "whooshing" sound and that the silver sphere was moving.

To her surprise, the image reminded her of a flying saucer. When she connected with the body feeling evoked by the image, she found that if the spaceship speeded up, she felt her neck pain lift up and out of her body as the spaceship lifted off. When I had her think about a recent spike of pain that occurred when she re-injured herself playing sports, she reported that when she thought about that incident, her neck pain returned with a vengeance (a 10 on a 10-point pain scale). I then asked her to test the strength of her flying saucer image, and when she brought that image into focus, her pain again lifted up as the spaceship gathered speed and started to lift off. When she examined her neck pain again, it was a 2 on the scale.

With practice, Maria found that the spaceship image, along with several other images, helped her regulate her cervical pain more effectively so that it was typically 3–4 points lower than usual. Whenever she had a flare-up, she found that she could use this image to begin to take her pain down more and more rapidly. At first this process required extended daily practice sessions. After several weeks, however, just thinking of the spaceship helped her keep her pain in a lower range.

Improve Your Results

Although we don't know precisely how and why imagery works, a few well-controlled research studies have yielded enough data to support some reasonable theories. Visual, auditory, and tactile imagery seems to originate in the cerebral cortex, the center of higher mental functions such as language, thinking, and problem-solving. Imagery involving taste, smell, and emotional experiences may arise in more primitive brain centers.

Experiments using PET (positron emission tomography) scans to monitor the brain during imagery exercises have demonstrated that the same parts of the cerebral cortex are activated whether people are *imagining* the object or event or *actually experiencing* it.[6] That means that picturing a visual image of a bridge activates the visual cortex in the same way as seeing the bridge directly. The more vivid the imagery produced, the closer to real impact it is believed to have. This is true whether the images are visual or constructed in another sensory modality.

Belleruth Naparstek, who has specialized in the use of imagery for many years, points out that guided imagery is especially useful for healing trauma. The traumatized brain tends to scan for nonverbal danger cues in the environment, rather than fixating on language and ideas. Individuals who suffer post-traumatic stress, which includes many chronic pain patients, experience heightened sensitivity in the areas of the brain that process emotions, sensations, and images, with a parallel shut-down in areas involved in language and cognitive processing. This post-traumatic sensitivity creates an ideal environment for the use of imagery, which can calm the hyperarousal in the brain so that higher thinking function can take place.[7]

I tell my pain clients that whether or not trauma was connected to the event or condition that originated their pain, having a chronic pain condition is *traumatizing* in and of itself. Many experts believe that trauma is one of the bridges between the multiple mechanisms of pain. A large percentage of chronic pain is the result of physical trauma such as muscular, tissue, joint, or nerve injury. In people whose pain did not clearly originate with physical trauma, post-traumatic stress disorder (PTSD) often can be diagnosed after a pain condition has progressed into chronic duration.

Unresolved shock resulting from many types of trauma that subsequently has been held in the body is also a major contributor to pain. Childhood physical and sexual abuse has a particularly high correlation with chronic pain conditions, for example. Shock can also include reactions to medical diagnoses of life-threatening illness such as a diagnosis of cancer or AIDS, accidents and injuries to the body, and responses to intrusive medical procedures, including surgery.

Since trauma has such a strong connection with chronic pain conditions, it is fortunate that imagery is such an effective intervention. Because the changes in the brain resulting from trauma impair language and organizational capacities, "talk therapy" alone is not likely to provide resolution of either the post-traumatic stress or the chronic pain condition. So, for a variety of important reasons, imagery is an important component of successful treatment of chronic pain. Unfortunately, many people feel discouraged about using imagery, a reaction that probably arises from one or more common errors involving its use.

Avoid Common Errors Made with Imagery

Error #1: Imagery is not successful unless it has at least some visual qualities. Even though we know that imagery can be constructed in any sensory modality, many people feel that they cannot image because they cannot construct visual images. In fact, effective imagery uses any or all of our *eight senses*: smell, taste, kinesthetic or tactile touch, vision, hearing, intuition, body felt sense, or proprioceptive sense.

Correction: Discover your primary imagery modality by completing the following brief exercise. Think of your favorite fruit. Notice what quality of the fruit impacts you the most—taste, smell, visual appearance, etc. Whatever sensory modality you led with to "find" the fruit, lead with that modality for the exercises that follow so that the images feel like yours rather than ones that you must conform to.

Error #2: It is the content of the image that is healing. Actually, it is the *impact* of the image on your mind/body/spirit and heart emotions that provides the healing effect. Virtually *any* image can have a positive impact. I once worked with a client whose healing image turned out to be a coffin! So open your mind to whatever your unconscious shares with you.

*Correction: Stay detached about the **content** of your imagery. Think for a moment about your area of pain. Focus outside the area or on the edge of it, if needed, to stay centered, rather than becoming overwhelmed. Challenge yourself to let a new image come forth that might give you some additional important information about your pain. There is NO way that your conscious thinking mind can know what that information will be or* *what form it will take. So no matter how ridiculous or inappropriate or unlikely an image the information might seem to you, practice being an open channel for whatever comes in, even if you can't assign a meaning. Make a note of that image or information here or in your pain notebook.*

Error #3: For imagery to be effective, you must use the same image consistently. The truth is that imagery is sometimes more effective if it moves and changes over time. Movement (or emanation) is the transformative quality that allows imagery to change as your experience does. If your image remains the same and you're getting good results, trust the stable form of your image. If your image changes, however, don't fight the change. Trust your imagination to create what is needed at any point in your healing process.

Imagery related to traumatic injury or persistent pain is often frozen or static, related to the freezing response of the nervous system. Allowing or helping an image move and change can help to unlock the freeze response. The use of **eidetic imagery,**[8] which you will practice next, is one way to help this movement along.

*Correction: Practice letting your imagery move. Choose one of your top five pain blockers. (We first explored these in Chapter One.) As you've been moving through the course, your top five pain blockers may have changed, so stay current and choose something that is working for you now. Create an image of one of the pain blockers and explore the feeling you get in your body when you tune into the image. Remember that you can get a "felt sense," a memory, or a mixed sensory image—neither content nor form is important. It is the **impact** on you that counts!*

After you have explored the image of taking a warm bath or watching your favorite TV program (just as examples), let the first image fade (if it helps, you can open your eyes to take a brief break), and then let another image of the same experience come into your mind. Spend a few moments exploring image #2 and find its connection to your body. Note

what is similar in the second image and the first image and what is dif-
ferent. Then let go of image #2 and let image #3 appear. Again, explore
the image and its connection with your body, noting similarities and dif-
ferences. Repeat this process to take the image further if you would like,
allowing images #4 and #5 to appear. Think about how your image devel-
oped during steps #1 through 5. What can you conclude about the trans-
formation of the image?

Remember that there are MANY ways to help imagery move. If
the eidetic imagery seems too complicated or does not appeal to you,
feel free to find your own method.

Exercise: Special Imagery Techniques with Pain
Conflict-Free Imagery[9]

This type of image is one that I have helped to pioneer in the last
five years. It was first explored in my earlier book, *Finding the Energy
to Heal*. The conflict-free image is based on the premise that all
human beings, regardless of their suffering, and regardless of the
degree or nature of their psychological or physical problems, have
an area of self-functioning that is without internal conflict.

This means that there are moments or longer periods of time during everyday life where there are no symptoms, no anxiety, depression, or distress, and yes, even no pain. If your pain feels constant, you
may reject this idea, perhaps under the mistaken impression that I am
describing a *positive* time of comfort and relief.

Conflict-free experiences are not necessarily positive, but they
are at least *neutral*. They signal a time of relative wholeness and
integration, which all of us have in some form, as long as we are
living beings with the potential of the breath of life that flows
through us.

The challenge is to find this conflict-free "zone" of experience
inside of us and to focus its energy on healing. One way of doing so

is to ask, "When am I most fully engaged in my life so that there is no inner conflict or resistance? When is a time when all of me participates in an experience that is so absorbing that I'm not aware of my pain or other symptoms?"

NOTE: For best results with the following exercise, approach this one step at a time with breaks if needed.

To explore the conflict-free image, take a few moments and quiet your mind and body using your preferred type of breath cycle. Add tension release or other skills you have learned to deepen your focus and relaxation. When you feel ready, begin to think about times in your day or week that you look forward to, times when you feel most like the way you want to feel more of the time and eventually all of the time, or even times that you do not dread. No matter what comes to your attention, accept it. [Remember, the content of the image is not what's important— it's the **impact** *of the image that matters.] Follow these steps to find your image:*

1. Identify a conflict-free experience. *Your conflict-free moment could be a brief time of quiet, alone time such as sitting and reading in your garden or your favorite corner in your living room with your cat in your lap or your dog curled up on the floor under your feet. It could be a time of social interaction such as playing a game with your children, grandchildren, or favorite nephews, or spending time with a close friend who makes you laugh no matter how bad you are feeling. If your pain has been at particularly high levels, perhaps it is even a time when you are asleep, just after you have taken your medication, or are soaking in the shower or tub.*

If you are having trouble identifying a conflict-free experience, spend a day "on the lookout," or ask someone who knows you well, when they experience you as being most without any conflict or pain.

2. Create an image that represents this experience. *Remember that it can be any kind of sensory image, a felt sense, even a thought. Lead with your primary sensory modality that you identified earlier in this chapter (in Correction #1 above).*

3. Try to connect all of your senses with this image—*taste, touch, smell, feel, appearance, texture, color, sound, intuition, felt sense, and proprioception (internal body sense in space).*

4. Make sure that the image evokes a conflict-free sensory connection. *Sometimes the connection with the conflict-free image can begin as positive, yet when you sit with it a few moments, it begins to feel more negative. A common example is an experience that you enjoyed in the past but are not able to enjoy now because of your pain symptoms. If sadness begins to come up or frustration, anger, irritability, or even despair or fear, set this aside, and after a break start again with step 1 above to find another image. If you persist, I guarantee you will find a conflict-free moment.*

5. Test the strength of the image *once you have found a wholly positive or at least a wholly neutral connection with an image.*

a. *If you are in significant pain of 5 or more, focus on the pain area and find out what happens to the conflict-free connection in your body. Pendulate back and forth between these two areas (see Chapters Two and Three) using the breath. Find out if you can create a body experience that stays at least neutral when you bring in the pain.*

b. *If you are fortunate enough not to be in pain at the moment you are practicing this, first focus on your conflict-free image. Then go back to a recent time of moderate pain (about a 4 to 6 on a 10-point pain scale). What happens when you pair the conflict-free image with your pain memory?*

c. *If the conflict-free image is overwhelmed by the pain memory, try to strengthen the conflict-free image by making it more vivid. Sometimes it helps to suggest to yourself that with the next breath in, you can "step into" the body that is in the conflict-free image and explore that possibility. Finding your pain-free body is a powerful experience.*

6. *If you are successful with step 5, practice finding the conflict-free image when your pain increases a little and is at 6 or below on your 10-point pain scale, for example. When you have good results with that, practice using your image when your pain is even higher.*

Exercise: **Circle of Pain Imagery**[10]

This type of imagery can help to contain or hold your pain so that it doesn't overwhelm you. You might want to read through the directions below a few times so that you can move through the exercise more easily, or perhaps record it in your own voice, or listen to it on an audio track.

Begin by sitting quietly after removing all distractions. Begin with your preferred type of breathing and, once you are starting to feel settled, add cue words such as "in" and "out" or "relax" . . . "now" when you are inhaling and exhaling. As you continue to focus on your breath, find a safe place in your body that seems or feels furthest away from the area of pain.

Next, add the tension-release method of relaxation (only if it is helpful to you), tensing the muscles in four to five areas of your body from head to feet, or sending the remaining tension or discomfort into your clenched fist or an object like a stone or marble. Hold your breath as you hold all the tension in your body and then when ready, let your breath and body go. . . . Repeat if needed. Then continue with the following script:

"Now that you have let go of some of your tension . . . scan your body for any aches, soreness, tightness, or discomfort . . . both physical and emotional. . . . When you are ready, begin to gather up the pain into a glowing, brightly colored circle. . . . When you have the circle in your

mind's eye, begin to play with the size, changing it. . . . Notice how the shadings and intensity of the color change as you make the circle larger . . . as you make the circle smaller. . . . Change the size and shape of the circle several times. . . . Allow it to become very large, gigantic, larger than your whole body . . . and then watch and feel as it shrinks down to a tiny dot. . . . Play with all of the possibilities of size, shape, and color. . . . Move the circle of pain out to the surface of your skin . . . and feel it resting gently now on the surface of your skin. . . . Notice the size and color as you imagine the circle beginning to float above the surface of your skin, floating up, up, and away . . . moving across the room . . . drifting through a window or even through a wall. . . . Imagine the circle of your pain . . . drifting out through your building and over the tops of the trees and other buildings and finally disappearing from sight. . . ."

Return to the feelings in your body, scanning both your upper and lower body . . . noticing any changes. . . . Knowing that each time you practice this, you will become more skilled at shifting your pain . . . and taking care of yourself . . . and as you take a few reenergizing breaths, come back to full awareness of the room around you . . . confident that whatever is right at this moment is unfolding for you . . . and will keep on unfolding long after you leave this exercise behind in the back of your mind.

Use Your Imagination to Prepare for Surgery or Other Medical Interventions

Most of us approach the idea of surgery with fear or denial. We may have heard so much about possible complications that we are terrified, or instead we've been told that a particular procedure is a "piece of cake." This type of unsolicited feedback makes it hard to develop a fresh, healthy, balanced perspective.

If you have minor anxiety about a medical procedure or other anxiety-producing event, this is normal and actually even desirable. It means that you are tuned into your reactions, which is far more helpful than being numb or "checked out." This self-awareness will allow you to work with and even change whatever negative reaction you are having.

In the case of a medical event, learn as much as you can about the particular medical procedure from your own doctor or surgeon. Then research further using the Internet or other resources. Be aware of the mental picture you may be forming as you study. What do you imagine will happen? What will it be like the night before? An hour before and after? A week after the event? Just let your own answers to these questions begin to form like a Polaroid print that gradually takes form.

Once you are aware of your responses, then ask yourself, "How do I want to be feeling the night before? An hour before? An hour after? A week later?" Allow yourself to make your own inner educational "film" so that you can coach yourself to feel as well as you possibly can within the reality that you are likely to feel some discomfort as part of the necessary healing process, much like a cut on your finger is tender while the skin is knitting back together again.

⌒ BOB

Bob was getting ready to have surgery on his wrist, which he had injured playing volleyball in an adult league. He had had the same procedure some years before and was scared that he would experience more pain because of his age (65) and because of intervening injuries over the years.

When we met, I suggested that Bob first imagine the best possible outcome. With some encouragement, he told me that he would spend the night before with friends who were supportive and encouraging, but not with his volleyball buddies, who had a tendency to "act like jocks" and minimize the possibility of any discomfort.

Bob envisioned that on the morning of the surgery, he would take his CD player to the clinic. He planned to listen to some of the recordings we had made to guide him in the use of positive imagery so that he could keep his mind focused on his body having the best possible experience—only as much discomfort and swelling that were necessary for healing, and the return of energy beginning later that same day. Bob imagined feeling hungry and thirsty a few hours after surgery so that his body systems could begin functioning as soon as possible, and he pictured taking a dose of pain medication to keep himself comfortable before his pain levels could go up after the anesthetic wore off.

By the day after surgery, he expected to be moving around normally, using a sling when his arm got tired, taking a nap, and enjoying his usual shower with his wrist bandage protected by plastic. Bob also planned to use that day and the next to catch up with fun reading and movies he wanted to watch. He recognized that his body needed to recover from the trauma of the surgery, and he wanted to help the recovery process along by keeping his mind in sync with his body.

Bob actually did quite well with this surgery. He later told me that being prepared through our imagery "dress rehearsal" had helped lower his anxiety and allowed him to stay more comfortable even than he imagined.

What is your positive fantasy of how your procedure will go? Record it in your pain notebook and remember that you can keep revising it right up until the time your procedure begins.

If you are not preparing for a medical event, apply this procedure to a social or other type of event that you dread attending because of your pain condition. Use your imagination to rehearse positive possibilities for reactions you want to develop.

How does your positive fantasy play out? Can you add or change any details to make it even more affirming?

Exercise: **Meet the Pain-Free Body That Is Alive and Well Inside You**

If you've been in pain for some time, you may have forgotten what it's like to feel pain-free, or even what it's like to experience pain that registers at only 2–3 on a 10-point pain scale. This exercise can help you recreate that body sense.

Take a few moments to get settled and start with your preferred type of breathing. Add any key words as you inhale or exhale. Then add your favorite type of enjoyable relaxation—tension release, the fist, the marble methods, or any other that works for you. Imagine that you are traveling across a bridge of time. The bridge can be an old covered bridge, a modern steel structure, or anything else you can create through your senses.

Imagine crossing the bridge between this moment now and back to the time when you first developed a pain condition. . . . As you move toward the end of the bridge, you may find yourself thinking and feeling more and more the way you did at that particular time . . . the time before the kind of pain you have now. As you step off the bridge, you may begin to remember some of the markers of that time in your life. . . . Maybe you can recall times when your body could move freely, when there were no restrictions in how and when you moved, when moving felt wonderfully free. . . . You may get some clues about how old you were, what was happening then or not happening, where you were, who was there. Give your body time to rediscover this experience, its sense of this pain-free time. With your next breath in, you can even imagine stepping into the body that was living that time, your time. As you exhale, allow your breath to move everywhere it could go then, as well as where it wants to flow now. Feel the relief, the release, the sense of spaciousness, along with any other aspect of your experience that you become aware of. Embrace all of this—then, now, all the spaces in between that are timeless and formless.

Maybe you can even feel a sense of surrender, of moving into your body that you can embrace fully through your eight senses. As you continue breathing, find out if you can get a sense of coming home to your body, to the pain-free self who has been waiting for you to find her or him again. Enjoy this reunion, feel the flow of it, and flow through the feel of it. And know that you can come back here again and again, whenever you form this intention. . . . And also know that each time will be different, depending on the moment you step off to cross the bridge of time travel . . . yet the experience of your body as home can be the same . . . more and more familiar to you with practice, more and more yours more of the time.

As you gradually become aware of your surroundings again, find out what parts of this pain-free body you can bring back with you. You might even want to find the bridge again and wander where you wandered a few moments ago . . . back into that sacred body space, just so you know you can find it again . . . back and forth, back and forth, until you're ready to stretch and move, all the way back on this side of the bridge again.

If you'd like to, take a few moments to savor this experience before you go on. Write about it in your pain notebook and think about how you would like to use this exercise again in the future.

SUMMARY: In this chapter, you learned about the eight senses, explored structured or guided imagery and how it is believed to work, and learned how to correct some common mistakes that are made with imagery. You had the opportunity to practice four imagery techniques for pain. They were the conflict-free image, the "circle of pain" technique, rehearsal for surgery or medical procedures, and connecting with the pain-free body. To end this chapter, you'll combine some of your growing skill with imagery with the foundational skills of the past three chapters to create a powerful resource to help you regulate your pain in several new ways.

Body Awareness Skill #4

IMAGINE Your Brain's Pain Relief Center and Your Body's Pain Solution

This exercise helps to regulate pain through imagery that is designed to turn on the mind-body connection by developing a sense of the brain's pain relief center. Because this imagery exercise can be long and somewhat detailed, you will want to set aside uninterrupted time to read the script below, record it in your own voice, or have a friend or loved one record it for you.

Keep in mind that this is a more structured script than the conflict-free imagery exercise you explored earlier in this chapter. Notice whether you have a more positive response to this kind of structured script than to the more open-ended kind.

Be open to which type of imagery is working better for you right now. If you aren't responding well to the script idea, you may want to save this exercise for a later time when your body's feedback lets you know that you are feeling more resonance.

Sit or lie comfortably with all distractions removed. Begin by focusing on your breath as it is moving through your body at this exact moment . . . shift gradually into your preferred type of breathing. . . . Repeat the breathing cycles until you feel you are beginning to settle in. Imagine your breath flowing into areas of tightness, pain, or discomfort. . . . Find the area in your body that seems or feels furthest away from the center of your pain at this moment. . . . Rest in that place for a few moments . . . appreciating the relief you can feel. . . .

If it's helpful to do so, tighten your muscles in your body . . . progressing from your feet gradually to your head (or reversing this sequence) . . . imagine that you can hold all the tightness and pain as you tighten your muscles . . . if you'd like, send all the discomfort into your tightened fist . . . or imagine or hold your marble and squeeze all the tension and pain into the marble. Hold all the tension and pain as you hold your breath . . . and when you are ready, let it all go. . . .

Now imagine that you will take a journey through your body . . . and that in order to do so, your adult body will begin shrinking and shrinking until it is less than an inch tall. . . . On the next breath in, imagine the **miniature you** moving in with your breath and moving through your body . . . traveling as you continue breathing through the airways in your body . . . moving easily with each breath until it arrives at the center of your pain. . . . You will discover that the miniature version of you has all the information and wisdom as your adult self, yet is not affected by the pain itself. . . . It's as if he or she is a powerful camera, searching the pain area . . . a curious explorer whose job it is to notice what is not as it should be and to send that information directly to you.

Take some time with this. What do you find? What does this area need? Consider all the possibilities . . . cooling . . . freezing . . . warming . . . repair of muscles or tissues . . . a special medication, perhaps, that will have a very specific and immediate effect—one that is superior to what you take now with NO side effects . . . only relief . . . what you have always wanted but did not think existed. . . . When you have reviewed all the information you want to gather for now, with the next breath in the mini-you can begin to travel again . . . moving through the air pathways . . . up toward the brain . . . through the diaphragm . . . the lungs . . . the upper chest . . . the windpipe . . . the throat . . . through the sinuses . . . behind the eyes . . . up to the forehead and into the front of the brain. . . .

When the mini-you arrives in the brain area, he or she will begin to look for the control room of the brain . . . and when the miniature self enters that room, he or she will see a huge array of switches and dials and screens and generators and equipment of all kinds. . . . Look around until the pain relief center is evident. Ask the mini-you to look until she or he finds what is needed at your pain center in the body. It may be a special coolant or medication that can be released through a tube that can be aimed right into the place that needs comfort the most. There will be a *switch or button to turn it on so that it starts flowing in just the right amount. . . . Turn on the switch and then set a timer if you'd like to. . . . Set the intensity of the healing intervention at a low number at first (for example at 2 out of 10 on a dial or gauge) until you can determine the effects . . . increasing only one number at this time so that you can find out how your body will receive what is given . . . bringing you a deep integration, which can only happen gradually with ease and comfort. . . .*

When everything is complete, the mini-you will begin to travel back down from the brain with the next breath out, again following the breath through its pathways . . . making its way through each exhalation . . . until it reaches the diaphragm, where it will rest until needed again. . . . Take your time and let your attention return fully to the room around you as your eyes open slowly. . . . Take a few moments to clarify what has happened and affirm your curiosity about how it might help you. . . . If you'd like, record some of your experience here on this page or in your pain notebook.

↩ SOPHIE

Sophie experienced severe facial pain due to TMJ (temporomandibular joint) dysfunction and several root canal surgeries. When she used imagery to tap into the brain's pain relief center, she added nitrous oxide, a drug that had helped her during her dental surgeries. She was able to turn the imaginary flow of nitrous oxide up high enough to increase comfort in her face and jaw. Since there were no side effects, she could use this technique whenever she liked. To enhance her results, she imagined a mask that dropped down, like oxygen masks on an airplane, whenever her pain became higher than 4 out of 10. She also added an imaginary irrigation system, something like the one in her garden, to circulate numbing liquid through her saliva.

The results Sophie obtained eventually enabled her to go back to work part-time and to very gradually decrease her pain medication.

Like any skill, the benefits of working with the brain's "Pain Relief Center" will develop over time. They may *not* be perfect or even very clear to you the first time or two. Many of my clients have taken several months of careful practice to create exactly the kind of healing effect they had been hoping for with this exercise. Eventually, with practice and time, the positive effects became strong enough and consistent enough to integrate and trust.

Many people who work effectively with this type of tool feel confident enough to gradually decrease or taper off their prescription and over-the-counter medication. As always, if you find yourself wanting to shift any medication you have been taking, make sure you have full medical support so you will have the best chance for *lasting* results.

CHAPTER FIVE

Mindfulness
Fill Your Mind with the Wisdom of Each Moment

Earlier in this book, we discussed the fact that all sources of pain send signals that travel down the same nerve pathways to the spinal cord and brain, regulated by the gating system in the spine's dorsal horn. Unresolved emotional suffering and grief have been identified by experts as important contributors to chronic pain, and these factors are explored in depth in Chapter Eight.

A less commonly identified root of chronic pain conditions is unresolved spiritual suffering. Persistent or chronic pain is an extraordinary event in life. It is powerful enough to force you to reexamine all your beliefs. Why is this happening to me? What does this pain mean? How do I endure it? At its worst, pain is persuasive enough to convince you that It is all-powerful, everlasting, out to you get you, and that there is no end to its power.

It is important not to allow pain to become a god. Fortunately, every spiritual tradition has ways to help you resurrect from the ashes of your pain. All paths to spiritual healing speak in some way of resurrection as transformation: the experience of being lifted up, transformed from extreme suffering and even death—and returned to our spiritual essence, or true self.

The good news is that although you may feel virtually imprisoned in the hell of uncontrollable pain as you read this paragraph, this is not the whole truth of your experience. When we muster enough courage to question, to really look at our pain, and stay present to our bodily experience of pain, we inevitably notice that our experience of pain shifts constantly, and that the body is amazingly resilient and filled with abundant healing resources to tap. We need only believe in these possibilities.

Most of us have heard the phrase that "pain is a great teacher." The metaphors used to describe pain—a wilderness, desert, black hole—are far from comforting or inspiring, however. At times when you are besieged by unrelenting pain, it may not feel helpful to consider that your pain can be the impetus for essential spiritual learning. Yet if you have focused significantly on the physical and emotional aspects of pain so far in your healing process, and feel that something is still missing, this might be a good time to consider how pain can provide an important opportunity for deeper healing and spiritual transformation. Perhaps you can envision this chapter as a type of pilgrimage to reclaim your spirit from pain.

The Spiritual Meaning of Pain

Authors from many spiritual traditions have written that "to live is to suffer" or that suffering is "the human condition." Yet we have a strong aversion to pain. We are quick to reach for medication if we develop a headache or muscle pain. Turning away from and numbing pain, while providing momentary comfort, may rob us of a deep dimension for healing in our lives.

Alexander Lowen, who created the body therapy method called *bioenergetics*,[1] a well-known model of physical healing, spent many bleak days of suffering in a World War II German prison camp. Yet he used this time as an opportunity to develop compassion for those who tormented him. By learning as Lowen did to find a way to use pain as a source of growth, we can cultivate more resilience instead of suffering and despair.

In her book *Turning Suffering Inside Out*, Darlene Cohen has written that the first step toward discovering the positive meaning of pain is to acknowledge your suffering—what it is costing you to live with a painful situation.[2] Your acknowledgement of pain and suffering will eventually allow you to explore all of your body experience and to enter the world of sensations, both positive and negative. She suggests that if you are in great pain most of the time, it becomes even more important to create a life of enjoyment and pleasure. Chronic pain can therefore propel us into greater determination to identify reliable sources of true comfort and to make a commitment to the new life we discover as we truly come to know our pain.

Author Gerald May, who wrote the classic *Grace and Addiction*, explored new ground in his last book, *Wilderness and the Spirit*,[3] written just before he died of cancer. During this last chapter of his life, he began to focus on the lessons he had learned from nature over the course of his life, and to blaze new trails in his wilderness experiences. Specifically, he emphasizes the wildness of nature and how it can reveal to us our own wildness. He expresses his regret that he spent so much of his psychiatric career counseling people to cope with their pain, which put them into an adversarial relationship with it. Instead, thanks to the wisdom gleaned from nature as his teacher, he advises us to be present to our pain and to discover the innate wildness that can be revealed.

You may already be aware of some of the deeper meanings and lessons of your physical pain. Does it force you to slow down in your life? Does it require you to focus more on your own needs and learn to care for the vulnerable parts of yourself? Does it remind you that there is unfinished emotional pain that you need to resolve? Is your pain an expression of your sense of spiritual disconnection, emptiness, or fragmentation and a longing for connection and wholeness? Or is pain (as Gerald May suggests) an invitation to wildness that defies our attempts to tame what is frightening? Pause for a few minutes to think about these possibilities.

Martha Beck recommends a daily practice to discover your deeper truth about pain.[4] She suggests starting with the general question, "What am I feeling?" and then welcoming whatever we become aware of—rage, resentment, jealousy, fear, and physical pain.

Out of this self-questioning may come the awareness of negative emotions, such as pain. We must next ask ourselves, "What hurts?" Make room for all your answers and let the feelings grow as big as they want to. Then ask, "What is the painful story I'm telling?" If you poke around with this third question, you will likely find your pain linked with past memories or fears of the future.

Follow with the fourth question: "Can I be sure my painful story is true?" Even if you have a knee-jerk "yes" response, sit with your story longer and you will begin to discover that your stories about pain are impossible to verify completely, because they are usually based on perceptions, not on facts. Beck's fifth question, "Is my story about pain working to really help me?" is followed by a sixth one, "Can I think of another story that might work better?"

This type of self-inquiry approach may be helpful to follow as you work your way through this chapter. Your pain notebook or journal can help to chronicle this aspect of your pain pilgrimage.

Again, skim through the chapter the first time to formulate your intentions and goals, then follow with a more thorough reading designed to master parts of the material that "speak" to you. Out of the vast treasury of wisdom and methods of spiritual exploration available from the great traditions, I have included a sample of the ones that I find particularly helpful in working with pain conditions. Although I do not advocate specific types of religious beliefs or practice, I have found that engaging in prayer or meditation that is meaningful for you will increase your chances of making a full recovery.

What Is Mindfulness?

The simplest way to define mindfulness is "non-judgmental attention to the ordinary in life." First and foremost is attention paid to the breath and to all the major senses, accepting what is seen, felt, tasted, touched, smelled, or heard. When you are *mindful*, you notice every aspect of the current moment without condemning, judging, interpreting, minimizing, demeaning, disliking, labeling, or comparing. As well-known Buddhist author and teacher Pema Chodron has written, rather than viewing ourselves as projects we need to improve, mindfulness is about "befriending who we are already."[5]

Gerald May notes that in our society, we spend great amounts of time and effort instructing our children to learn to concentrate on one task at a time, thereby teaching them to tune out everything else around them. Unfortunately, this can result in a "tunnel vision" which robs us of our natural connection to all living things, and to the symphony of sounds, tastes, smells, and other sensory delights.

The two main tools of mindfulness are *attention* and *intention*. Attention requires the development of what is called "beginner's mind," the willingness to begin again and again as your linear mind becomes distracted when thoughts intrude. Mindful attention is like holding a raw egg; if you grasp it too tightly, it will crack; if you hold it too loosely, it will drop and break.

Yet even if you develop a balanced mind-full attention toward your everyday life, without positive *intention*, this will be a mechanical process. If your *intention* is to be loving and compassionate toward yourself through every aspect of your experience, however, eventually you will cultivate inner calm and spaciousness about yourself, your pain, and your life. It is important that your intention be to open to all aspects of aliveness, to be fully present with the greater Presence of Spirit as God, the Buddha, Allah, or whatever divine image is central to your spiritual beliefs and faith. The technique you will explore next will help you deepen further your mindfulness of body presence.

Mindfulness Meditation

Jon Kabat-Zinn is one of the first medical experts to determine that the study of meditation and mindfulness is an effective antidote to chronic pain. Kabat-Zinn points out that many people have the attitude that their bodies are machines; therefore, their approach to resolving pain is to find a professional who will serve as a mechanic and "fix it." Since the body is NOT merely a machine, however, the "fix it" approach is very seldom effective. Because there is always a "mind" component to pain, it is far more effective to mobilize the resources of the mind to modify the perceptions of pain, thereby closing the gates and shutting pain down.

Kabat-Zinn's research shows conclusive evidence that the pain patients who are taught and who practice mindfulness meditation in his clinic have made four to ten times greater improvement than pain patients who were receiving powerful medical interventions exclusively.[6] He concludes that engaging in mindfulness meditation practice, *in addition to* receiving medical treatments, results in positive changes that might not occur with medical treatment alone.

Exercise: The Body Scan

This is among the most useful mindfulness techniques for dealing with persistent and chronic pain. Bringing true healing to your body requires that you learn to be mindful of many aspects of your body's experience at any given moment.

Start by clearing your surroundings of distractions and take about 10 minutes to practice this method. You may want to make an audiotape of your own voice moving through the directions below. Be sure to leave plenty of time after each suggestion on the recording to focus on your experience.

Find a comfortable position so that all of your body feels supported. Close your eyes (if that is comfortable) and feel how your belly expands as you breathe in and sinks down as you breathe out.

Bring your attention to either the top of your head or the bottom of one of your feet. While continuing to focus on your breathing, notice that particular part of your body, imagine that you are breathing into that area of the body, and rest in stillness for a couple of breaths before moving on. If your thoughts wander, gently return them to your breathing and the particular part of your body you are exploring. When it is time to move on, let go of it completely. Even if your pain gets a little more intense, or does not seem to change at all, move on to the next part of your body, directing your attention and your breath into that new area, and gradually moving from your head down to your feet, or from your feet to the top of your head.

It is helpful to notice any thoughts or reactions you are having to your body or to your pain. Notice these non-judgmentally. Do not become attached to either success with the scan or to an apparent lack of progress.

If your body pain becomes so intense that you cannot maintain a focus, let go of your intention to scan, shut off the tape if you are listening to one, and focus directly on the pain. Keep your intention focused on learning about your pain and from your pain, not on getting rid of it. Open to the pure sensations, noting them, breathing with them. Keep practicing, bringing yourself back from distraction, staying with a body area, then moving on to the next.

Develop a perspective of witnessing, of neutral observation throughout. As your body scan comes to a close, tune into the experience of being in the present moment, without having to resolve problems or correct bad habits. Try to sense yourself as pure "being." Remember that success with mindfulness involves patience and gentleness and lovingkindness toward yourself.

When you finish the body scan, you may want to record some notes about your experience here, in your pain notebook, or on a special chapter bookmark that summarizes your discoveries.

The Power of Now

In part, mindfulness is effective because we learn the positive effects of focusing fully on the present moment. Author Eckhard Tolle, who has written *The Power of Now* and *Practicing the Power of Now*, discusses mindfulness in a compelling way that helps us experience and understand this truth.

Tolle writes of entering the NOW: "With the timeless dimension comes a different kind of knowing, one does not 'kill' the spirit that lives within every creature and every thing. A knowing that does not destroy the sacredness and mystery of life but contains a deep love and reverence for all that is. A knowing of which the mind knows nothing."[7]

Tolle suggests that if you have difficulty being present in the NOW directly, start by observing the habitual ways your mind wants to escape from the present moment. Usually, we imagine the future as either better or worse than the present time. *It can be helpful to notice how often your attention strays to the past or future.* Presence, in Tolle's view, is the key to freedom. You can only be free now in this moment. Remind yourself that the present moment is all you ever have. Practice saying "yes" to the present moment.

Exercise: **Be in the Now with Your Senses**

Read the following practice exercise through once then read it a second time, phrase by phrase. Pause after each sentence and *experience* what you are reading.

*Be fully where you are right now. Look around you. Just look; don't inter-
pret or judge. See the light, shapes, colors, textures. Point these out to
yourself: "I see the surface of the desk, the piles of paper," and so forth.
Be aware of the silent presence and your felt sense of each object. Be
aware of spaciousness that allows everything to be.*

*Listen to sounds; don't judge them. Listen to their different qualities
and to the silence that lies underneath the sounds that you hear in this
moment.*

Touch anything. Feel and acknowledge its Beingness.

*Watch the rhythm of your breath. Feel the air flowing in . . . and the
air flowing out. Feel the life energy inside your body. Allow everything
to be exactly as it is, inside you and around you. Allow the "Is-ness" of
all things. For this brief moment, accept things just as they are. Move
deeply into the Now.*

*As you enter this now moment more fully with your senses, you can
leave behind the deadening world of the thinking mind that can drain your
life energy, just as it is slowly poisoning and destroying the Earth. You are
now awakening out of the dream of time into the present, the now.*

If you had difficulty with this simple exercise based on Tolle's work[8]
or need more practice, here is another way of training your mind to
be aware of the present moment experienced through your senses.

Exercise: **Sensory Awareness Training**

This is also called the "4-3-2-1 exercise."[9] And you will soon discover why. Since this method can be quite challenging for some
people, stay aware of your body's "yes and no" responses to determine whether this is a good fit. After several practice sessions, you
should notice an expansion of your sensory awareness in the current moment.

Begin with your external awareness of four sights, four sounds, and four feelings:

a. *Clear away any distractions for the next 10 minutes or so. Take a moment to sit or lie comfortably, eyes open with a soft visual focus. Notice four things you can see without moving your head. Tell yourself inwardly what these are: I see _____, _____, _____, and _____.*

b. *Then become aware of four sounds you can hear. Tell yourself what these sounds are: I hear _____, _____, _____, and _____.*

c. *Be aware of four things you can touch or feel: Four things I can feel right now are _____, _____, _____, and _____.*

Then shift to three things you can see, three sounds you hear, three things you can touch or feel. Name those: "Three things I can see right now are _____, _____, and _____."

Repeat with three things you can hear, then touch or feel.

*Next notice two sights, sounds, and feelings. It is OK to repeat ones you have noticed before **as long as they are true for you in this moment also.***

Finally, finish with one sight, one sound, and one feeling.

Then allow your eyes to close and begin with four internal images you can see. [HINT: The internal sensory experiences are more difficult because they may be unfamiliar to you. Do the best you can and be willing to stop if you become stuck. This gets easier with practice—remember that this is a training exercise. Also remember that it really doesn't matter if what you "see" is visual, or if what you feel is kinesthetic, proprioceptive, or the felt sense.] Continue with four internal sounds you can hear, four internal sensations you can feel.

Repeat with three internal images, sounds, and sensations. Then with two internal images, sounds, and sensations. Finish with one inner image, sound, and sensation.

Take a few moments to record your experience here if that is helpful to you. What was the easiest sense for you? The hardest? How did you feel at the end of the exercise?

Exercise: **Finding Inner Strength**[10]

There are many paths to discover and experience the spiritual self. In working with chronic pain, I have found that many clients find it helpful to connect with aspects of the spirit through a simple exercise designed to access the energy of Inner Strength.

Inner strength is conceptualized as a combination of courage, perseverance, determination, resolve, and grit. Inner strength is a conflict-free energy in the personality that every person possesses, believed to be related to the survival instinct. What follows is a script that can be used to access inner strength. Read it through first before you listen to an audio track (maybe recorded in your own voice). Be sure to leave space during the pauses for you to explore your inner experience. Feel free to change any of the script so that it can resonate more fully for you.

I would like to invite you to take a special journey within yourself to the center of your being . . . to a place that is very quiet . . . peaceful and still. And when you are in that place inside, it's possible for you to find an important aspect of yourself—an energy we will call your "Inner Strength."

Inner Strength has been with you since before you were born. It connects you to the life force in the universe. It's that energy inside you that has helped you to survive during difficult times . . . to overcome many, many obstacles in your past . . . just as it is the energy that helps you now to overcome obstacles . . . whether you have been aware of it or not. . . . Take a little time now to get in touch with that energy. You can notice what images . . . or feelings . . . or body sensations . . . even colors and symbols . . . come to you through your inner mind. Be open to whatever you receive.

*I'm going to count now from 5 to 1, and each number can guide you deeper inside toward the center of your being. 5 . . . Beginning to follow your breath so that each time you breathe in, you become more aware of the life force energy flowing through you. . . . 4 . . . This is the energy that connects you with all the wisdom and strength in the universe, with that which has come before you and all that will come after you. . . . 3 . . . This is an energy that is afraid of nothing and of no one. . . . 2 . . . This is an energy that has only and always your best interests and your deepest needs as its motivation. . . . 1 . . . When you are connected with this energy you may experience a feeling of **oneness** with yourself and with the world around you.*

Take a few moments now to connect with your Inner Strength . . . Opening to whatever you begin to find . . . Like an open channel, just let whatever is connected to your Inner Strength appear: body sensations, imagery, an inner voice, a past memory, symbols, emotional feelings, colors, a presence, or any combination of these. Explore whatever you find inside now . . . you might want to communicate with Inner Strength . . . to find out what it has done for you in the past and what it is willing to do for you now. . . . You'll find that you can communicate easily . . . without any need for words. . . . Be sure to arrange an easy way for you to find Inner Strength whenever you want or need to . . . perhaps by calling forth these images, feelings, or whatever you have found. . . .

As you say goodbye to Inner Strength for now, you know that you will meet again whenever and wherever you like . . . indirectly or directly . . . accidentally or on purpose . . . and as I count from 1 to 5, you can begin to bring some of this experience back with you. 1 . . . Feeling more confident now that you have the resources you need inside you that will help you resolve the challenge of pain . . . 2 . . . have additional energy to help you take the next steps forward in your healing . . . 3 . . . noticing new feelings of calm and well-being . . . 4 . . . more possibilities of strength now that will be growing inside you . . . and 5 . . . as you get ready to

*move and stretch and to open your eyes, the more confidence you feel
that you can use these resources you have found to be in touch with your
inner strength as a guide and an inspiration . . . taking your time to complete whatever is necessary . . . so that this experience can be fully useful to all of you. . . . Coming back now to your full waking self.*

*Take a few minutes and explore your experience with Inner Strength.
For best results, practice once a day for several days. Then, when you
are confident of your ability to find your inner strength energy, practice
without the script or audio to see if you can invoke inner strength in any
way to help you cope with worries or fears related to your pain condition.
What happens? If you'd like, record your results.*

Exercise: **Practice Lovingkindness (*Metta*) Meditation**

The basis of spirituality is **love.** Many spiritual writers from diverse
traditions have emphasized the belief that the deepest happiness we
experience in life is not related to how much we possess but to discovering the capacity to love and to have a loving relationship with
God, ourselves, and all of life.

"Metta," an ancient Buddhist lovingkindness practice that originated more than 2,500 years ago, offers a way to cultivate lovingkindness in oneself and toward others. The best method is to
repeat the practice of *metta* for 15–20 minutes once or twice a day
(you might want to start with 5 minutes) over a period of several
weeks or even months. Some people find it strange and even irri-
tating to direct wishes for love to themselves. If you find yourself
feeling frustrated, practice being aware of any feelings or reactions
that come up. Although *metta* meditation is ultimately used to direct
lovingkindness toward others, the emphasis is first placed on learning to send and receive *metta* for yourself. The belief is that you cannot truly love others until you have learned to love yourself.

To practice lovingkindness meditation,[11] practice saying the following phrases inwardly to yourself, much like repeating a mantra. Let feelings and images arise to help you begin to feel the impact of the messages. You might want to imagine yourself as a young child or at a different age, for example, or being in a different setting. Play with the words and the images until you find the exact words that seem to release feelings of love and compassion toward yourself that you can begin to really feel.

May I be filled with lovingkindness.
May I be well.
May I be peaceful and at ease.
May I be happy.

Even if you don't feel the impact of these words, continue practicing anyway. The power of positive **intentions** toward yourself, even if you don't feel them, will eventually pay rich dividends. Some people find it helpful to combine these phrases with walking meditation so that the rhythmic movement of the body and breath coordinate to make more of a connection to the words than can be done while sitting. If you try this, experiment with repeating each phrase on an in-breath/out-breath cycle.

After you have directed these messages to yourself and have started to feel more loving and compassionate toward yourself, you can take further steps. [Do not rush this process. It is not advisable to move on to sending messages of lovingkindness to others until you are responding positively to yourself first.]

Now, direct the phrases to someone who has been a helpful teacher or mentor to you. Translation of the Pali word "metta" is "benefactor." Think of someone who has had a big positive influence on you. Create an image or sense of your benefactor or mentor and hold the image in your mind's eye while repeating the following phrases inwardly:

May you be filled with lovingkindness.
May you be well.

May you be peaceful and at ease.
May you be happy.

Again, practice long enough to receive positive results. Then add images or thoughts of all your loved ones. Direct these phrases of lovingkindness now to those you love, either individually or as a group:

May you be filled with lovingkindness.
May you be well.
May you be peaceful and at ease.
May you be happy.

After this, you can experiment with neighbors, strangers, and acquaintances, then beings everywhere. Direct these phrases toward them. Finally, practice creating imagery or thoughts of people you find very difficult in your life. Direct these same phrases now to them.

↩ SYLVIA

Sylvia had never had much success with meditation because she could not sit still without becoming increasingly uncomfortable and even irritable. When we discussed the practice of *metta*, Sylvia decided to try this form of meditation while walking in the grassy area around her house. Over time, she evolved the following rhythmic mantra:

"May I walk through this day with ease and well-being,
May I walk through this day with peace and joy."

She repeated these phrases in tune with her walking and added similar ones for others she wanted to bless with *metta*:

"May you move through this day with ease and well-being,
May you move through this day with peace and joy."

If sitting meditation is not comfortable for you, you may want to try Sylvia's solution by adding the positive intentions to walking meditation. If you do not notice any immediate feelings of well-being, keep in mind that this entire subtle process may take several weeks; as it was originally taught in Tibet, *metta* meditation required seven years to master!

Prayer and Remote Healing

Larry Dossey, MD, a noted physician in the area of mind-body processes, has researched the effects of prayer on healing. He discusses many interesting studies. One of them, conducted by Herb Benson at Harvard Medical School (who also developed the relaxation response discussed in Chapter Three), studied the effects of different types of prayer such as the use of one word, like a mantra, a phrase, or the first line of prayer such as the Lord's Prayer. Benson found that all traditions of prayer were helpful in stimulating positive effects in the body, and that prayer consisting of words that were meaningful to patients had the best chance of helping with this process.

Perhaps one of the most well-known studies on prayer was conducted by a cardiologist, Dr. Randolph Byrd,[12] in a San Francisco coronary care unit of 393 patients. Half were assigned to a group whose members were prayed for by a remote prayer group, and half of the patients were not prayed for. The remote prayer groups were given the names of the patients and their diagnoses but were not told how to pray for them, only that they should pray every day. Patients in the prayed-for group each had five to seven people in different locations praying for them. The heart patients who were prayed for surpassed those who were not prayed for in several important ways: 1) They were five times less likely to require antibiotics; 2) They were three times less likely to develop pulmonary edema; 3) None required intubation; and 4) None died.

Only a few studies have been conducted specifically with pain. One of the best of these explored how religious and spiritual factors are related to daily positive emotional moods and pain reduction. Higher levels of faith successfully predicted greater reduction in pain, and a combination of faith and social support predicted greater reductions in both pain and negative moods.

The message is that if you believe prayer can help you heal your pain, it will. You might want to conduct your own study about how different forms of prayer might be helpful for you with your pain. Various types of prayer have been found to be effective for many healing situations, including the practice of asking for a specific healing outcome, expressing faith in the help you will receive, and asking for and granting forgiveness of self and others, especially family members. Experiment with different types of prayer and record your pain levels to see if you notice any interesting patterns.

If you find that your spiritual faith is shaky as you work through this chapter, you may want to talk with a spiritual director or psychotherapist who is experienced in working with spiritual issues to help you strengthen your relationship to the divine. Pain of long duration can challenge even the strongest spiritual faith. My experience is that it is almost impossible to heal persistent or chronic pain *by yourself*. This truth speaks to the necessity of finding supportive community and a regular prayer or meditation life.

As a final note, many people find it difficult to pray because they aren't sure how to go about it. Brother David Steindl-Rast, Benedictine monk and author, proposes that prayer is gratitude, about life lived in fullness. When we are awakened to full life in the divine, our eyes can be opened to the gifts we receive each day. Even when we struggle with pain, we can come fully alive if we are open to the surprise gifts that come our way. Brother David invites us to true mindfulness through a life grounded in gratitude. He invites us to "an attitude of gratitude."

As a daily practice, challenge yourself to find new experiences that you have never felt grateful for. If we look "through the eyes of our heart," as Steindl-Rast suggests,[13] we can see the wonders of a cloud formation, hear an exquisite bird song, notice the perfection of a sweet and beautiful blossom, and celebrate the smiling eyes of a loved one. Gratitude helps us focus on all that we are given, rather than the losses and pain we suffer.

SUMMARY: This chapter presented several approaches to the practice of mindfulness, a practice of meditation and awareness that has been highly successful with chronic pain and other health conditions. First, you considered the meaning of pain and read a brief presentation on mindfulness. You practiced the body scan as a mindfulness technique. You then explored two sensory-awareness training approaches. One was related to Tolle's work, designed to help you be present in the moment with your senses; the second was the 4-3-2-1 exercise, which helped you develop external and internal sensory awareness. Finally, you learned about Inner Strength as an aspect of spirit related to the life force in the universe, explored the Tibetan meditation practice for developing lovingkindness, and considered the power of personal prayer. This chapter closes with a mindfulness exercise that brings together many of these techniques and concepts.

Body Awareness Skill #5

MINDFUL Meditation:
Radical Awareness for the Self-Treatment of Pain

Begin with your preferred type of breathing. As you feel your body beginning to settle, allow yourself to become aware of your full experience in this moment.... Be aware of whatever you are feeling in your body, whatever you are thinking, any emotions that are present, and any images or other types of sensations.... Accept and acknowledge each one.... If it is helpful, conduct a body scan (described earlier in this chapter) to find all the important parts of your experience.

When your awareness feels full, gather together all the things that you have noticed with great kindness and gentleness toward yourself. [Example: "I accept with kindness and gentleness that right now I am feeling tightness in my throat, that my mind is thinking negative thoughts about how this won't work for me, that my hands are relaxed and warm, and that my arm and wrist are throbbing and aching."] As you take the next breath in, hold all of this in your awareness along with your breath, and when you are ready, let all of this go as you exhale.

On the next breath in, step into a new moment as if for the very first time with beginner's mind. Be open to what you may find in this new moment and explore it. [Again, use a body scan if that is helpful.] Name for yourself silently all that you are aware of in your body, mind, and heart until your awareness is full. Then gather all the aspects of your awareness together with great compassion and lovingkindness toward yourself. Hold these in your awareness as you hold your breath. When you are ready, let it all go. . . .

Then on the next breath in, step into another new moment with beginner's mind. Again, give yourself permission to be open to whatever you become aware of in your body, your emotions, your mind's eye, your thoughts, your other senses. Acknowledge each aspect of your experience and name it for yourself until your awareness feels full. Then gather all that you have noticed with great compassion and kindness toward yourself. Hold these in your awareness as you hold your breath. When you are ready, let it all go as you exhale. . . .[14]

Continue this practice for 5–10 cycles. What do you notice? How has your experience shifted from the beginning of the exercise to the end? How can you use this awareness practice to work in a more mindful way with your pain condition? Record your ideas in your pain notebook or on a chapter bookmark.

CHAPTER SIX

Energize
Find the Energy to Heal

The emerging fields of energy medicine and energy psychology offer promising new possibilities for treating successfully and efficiently many clinical and health problems, including chronic pain, that do not respond to mainstream interventions.[1]

This chapter will give you an opportunity to explore your energy system. You will learn how strengthening and rebalancing this system can help other types of pain treatment work more effectively. For many people, studying energy approaches requires a huge shift in their beliefs about healing. We have been taught to rely on the science of medicine, yet that science has not gone far enough in helping us solve our evolving pain epidemic. I invite you to keep an open mind as you study the material in this chapter. The goal is not to reject Western medicine but to balance what works best for you from traditional medicine with the hopeful possibilities found in alternative healing. Skeptics[2] are welcomed. You'll be in good company!

Alternative healing methods such as acupuncture, Reiki, qi gong, and yoga are believed to work because they stimulate what the Chinese call *qi* and the Hindus have termed *prana*. These terms refer to subtle life-force energies that shape, influence, and support the physical body. From the Eastern perspective, harmony in the mind-body system is based on energy flow and transformation.

Disharmony and imbalance can significantly block transformative energy flow inside an organ system, within a meridian network or energy pathway, through an energy station known as a *chakra*, or in the energy field surrounding the body. Energy barriers can originate from unresolved trauma, prolonged stress reactions, biological depression, nutritional deficiencies and food allergies, environmental toxins, and many other factors. Learning how to treat these kinds of energy imbalances can relieve stress and help correct symptoms of imbalance that include chronic pain.[3]

How Energy Therapies Can Help with Pain Relief

There are several benefits of using energy methods to help with pain relief:

1. Energy methods can help us deal with the complexity of pain, health problems, and trauma without adding more complexity. Because they are simple to learn and practice, they can be used easily with other methods without negative reactions. Pain pioneers Melzack and Wall believe that the future of pain relief lies in the effective use of multiple therapies. This is a principle that I have called the "AIDS Cocktail" approach to pain treatment (see Chapter One).

This term refers to how the spread of the AIDS epidemic was finally slowed. Because no one drug proved significantly effective in the battle against this disease, researchers combined medications to create a powerful, synergistic "cocktail" that is still used to treat the disease. With chronic or persistent pain problems, I've had the greatest success using different combinations of the methods included in this book, adding them in slowly and gradually until we find a "tipping point" that tips the scales away from unrelenting pain and gains momentum toward comfort, relief, and balance.

Benefit: Energy therapies are easy to learn, highly portable, and can be combined with many other therapies including somatic therapies, psychological therapies, physical therapies, and drug therapy to provide a multi-pronged approach.

2. Even if the root cause of your pain cannot be repaired (for example, in the case of degenerating spinal discs), much can be done to relieve your suffering. There are many cases of individuals who begin to feel so confident about regulating their discomfort that their experience of pain drops significantly, even if the condition that causes the pain has not changed.

Benefit: Energy therapies help relieve negative emotional reactions related to pain, especially anxiety and panic, along with the beliefs that create suffering and block healing efforts. You will learn several of these methods during this chapter.

3. Energy methods are consistently beneficial in helping to treat various types of stress, including post-traumatic stress that can worsen pain conditions.

Benefit: Unlike many other therapies, energy methods do not carry the risk of increasing pain when the focus is on past trauma because you don't have to focus on distressing trauma details. The worst that can happen when you try energy techniques is **nothing**—*that is, you may not have a significant reaction to the techniques in either a positive or negative direction.*

Energize, Don't Catastrophize!

When you have chronic pain, one of the common reactions you may encounter is connected to your own fears. When your pain increases suddenly and you cannot identify a reason or trigger for this change, a natural response is to feel scared and out of control. These types of fears can lead you to "catastrophizing" about your pain levels. If you are catastrophizing as a coping mechanism, your inner dialogue might go something like this: "Oh no. This pain increase proves how miserable my life is becoming. . . . Pretty soon I'm going to be in this pain all the time. I will run out of things that can help, and then what will I do?"

You are probably already aware of how destructive this type of negative thinking can be. The problem is, how do we stop catastrophizing? Although there are many ways to interrupt this type of thinking pattern,[4] one of the easiest strategies is to focus your mental attention on increasing positive energy and vitality levels. The following exercise will teach you several ways of doing just that.

Exercise: **The Three Boosters**

One of the first principles emphasized in using energy techniques is the importance of preparing for any treatment by creating a positive energy field. Although there are many methods used to achieve this, I have developed a streamlined method called "The Three Boosters."[5]

1. First, drink lots of water to get your energy moving. The energy we are working with is the body's electromagnetic energy. What is the best conductor of electrical energy? Of course you know—water! Make sure you have plenty of water ready before you try any protocol. Drinking water is believed to unlock the freeze response and keep the energy system flowing at its optimal level.

2. Next, balance the energy system by minimizing the danger of too much energy. When we experience severe pain or high stress, we may be in a situation where too much energy is trying to flow through our energy meridians or energy pathways. You can easily feel this happening if you experience panic or intense fear. If the energy system becomes chronically disorganized (through trauma hyperactivation, for example), symptoms can develop that lead to serious imbalance in mental clarity, resilience, and overall health functioning.

One of the conditions related to energy disorganization is that the nervous system scrambles and misinterprets nerve impulses. This has important implications for chronic pain conditions, so it is crucial to correct for "overenergy," even if you don't think you have this problem!

The condition of "overenergy" is believed to be related to the fight/flight/freeze response of trauma. An alarm has been sounded, at conscious or unconscious levels, and the brain, nervous system, and major organ systems respond by turning up the intensity for all major functions—heartbeat, respiration, blood pressure, and so on.

Correct for "overenergy," the stress condition that exists when too much energy, usually triggered by the fight/flight/freeze response, tries to flow through the meridians. Practice the following exercise, which may appear somewhat quirky at first until you experience its benefits. Most people experience a dramatic calming or settling response in just a few seconds.

- *While sitting or lying down comfortably, place your left ankle over your right;*
- *Extend your arms in front of the body with **backs** of your hands touching each other;*
- *Cross your right hand and arm over your left and clasp fingers together;*
- *Fold your arms and rest hands comfortably under chin on your chest;*
- *Rest your tongue against the palate behind the top of your front teeth; [Yes, I agree. This is a strange exercise!]*
- *Breathe for 1–2 minutes with both eyes and mouth closed.*

What was this experience like for you? Practice this approach whenever you feel "spaced out," overstressed, or experience a "pain spike." This is also a stand-alone rapid stress-reduction technique—one of my favorites!

If this causes any discomfort in your arms, hands, or legs, please modify your pose. For example, crossing your arms across your chest can bring the same benefits, and crossing your ankles in the opposite direction (right over left) or imagining that you are crossing them in either direction is another modification.

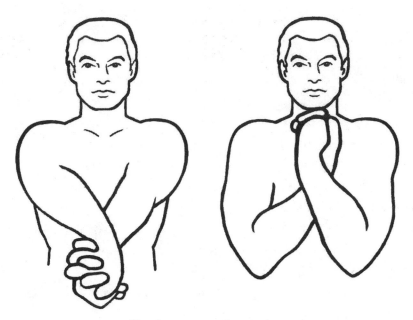

The Overenergy Correction

3. Create a positive energy field by correcting reversals. Although there are many ways to create a positive energy field, one of the best methods is to correct for what are called *psychological reversals*. Reversals refer to situations where the outcome is the opposite of the intention. All of us experience this. We want to lose weight and yet our efforts tend toward the opposite direction. We want to be successful at work and yet somehow, we don't progress. Reversals are subtle disturbances in the energy system that can result in an inner struggle or battle.

In order to *reverse* the course of a pain condition, it is important to know what inner conflicts may be preventing you from making use of the tools that could help you find the "tipping point" that can lead to a life where pain is no longer in control. Although there are many ways of finding and detecting these inner obstacles,[6] working with the form they take in the energy system is highly efficient and, unlike other approaches, will not add the risk of stirring up reactions that can create other obstacles to your progress.

This technique works to create a positive energy field by correcting for common reversals found in relation to most symptoms, including chronic pain. We use a specific kind of affirmation to make these corrections, which leads us to working with negative beliefs that often block us from progressing, as well as creating subtle energy disturbances.

A word here about affirmations: Although positive affirmations have been used commonly as part of various healing approaches, many people are bothered by saying them. Energy affirmations are somewhat different. With these, you will be describing *the undesirable problem you want to eliminate exactly as you experience it.* At the same time you will be affirming unconditional love for yourself by stating the phrase, "I deeply and completely love and accept myself." If this wording does not resonate or feel true, however, please change the language so that it *is* true for you. For example, you may substitute statements like "I want to be able to love and accept myself," "I know I am doing my best to heal," or "I believe I deserve to feel better."

Rub or hold a sensitive point on your left chest.[7] To find this point, first find your collarbone. Feel along the bone at your neckline and you will notice that there are small notches on either side of the midline of your body. Find the point that is 1 inch below the collarbone notch at either side of the midline and 3–4 inches toward the shoulder (almost to the shoulder crease). If you are worried about finding the right spot, use several fingers. Sometimes this spot is a little tender or sore.

Say the following affirmation out loud (this is to involve the energy vibrations of your voice) three or more times while stimulating this point on your left chest. It's also OK to rub these points on both sides of your chest. You can rub gently, tap with your fingers, or touch lightly while breathing.

First repeat the general affirmation out loud three times: "I deeply and completely love and accept myself **even though I have this pain**" (or feeling, symptom, reaction, etc.). Remember to use whatever words resonate fully for you at the time you are doing this exercise. You may want to use a more general statement following the affirmation, such as "I deeply and completely love and accept myself **even with all my problems and limitations.**"8

After you have repeated this general affirmation three times, continue stimulating this same left chest point while repeating some of the affirmations listed below designed to correct other negative beliefs or conflicts you may want to be free of. Each of these may be said aloud once after completing the general affirmation. Try all of them at first, but in future practice repeat the ones that seem or feel most true for you.

- "I deeply and completely love and accept myself even though . . . I'm afraid I can't change my pain problem."

- "I deeply and completely love and accept myself even though . . . I believe it's impossible to get over or resolve this pain problem."

- "I deeply and completely love and accept myself even though . . . I feel guilt and shame about having this pain problem."

- "I deeply and completely love and accept myself even though . . . I believe there's something wrong with me that I can't resolve this pain. . . ."

- "I deeply and completely love and accept myself even though . . . I am scared that I will never be free of this pain."

- "I deeply and completely love and accept myself even though . . . I may not feel ready or willing to do what it takes to resolve this pain problem."

- "I deeply and completely love and accept myself even though . . . I believe I don't deserve to get over this pain condition."

- *"I deeply and completely love and accept myself even though . . . I believe (or part of me believes) it might be unsafe to resolve this pain."*

Notice which ones resonate most strongly and mark them on this list. Please add any other limiting beliefs that you think may be blocking your ability to move forward in resolving your pain. You might want to use this formula for creating new affirmations just by changing the final phrase:

"I deeply and completely love and accept myself, even though I

_____."

[Fill in your statement of the problem.]

Although these affirmations are deceptively simple, they seem to correct energy reversals. Since reversals involve unconscious resistance to a desired outcome such as pain relief or anxiety reduction, perhaps the statements work because they address and accept these hidden conflicts at an energetic level.

Working with Your Pain Triggers

Now that you've rebalanced your energy system and created a positive energy field by correcting for reversals, you are ready to try out "an energy protocol," which is the term for a step-by-step plan designed to help you shift or relieve your pain. First we will use a simple technique that can be very effective with *pain triggers*—these are circumstances that can provoke a sudden increase in your pain. Triggers are different for each person but usually include experiences that are physically or emotionally stressful or some combination of both. They may or may not be related to past trauma, but often are.

Exercise: **The TAT**

We will start with the **TAT (Tapas Acupressure Technique)**[9] developed by acupuncturist Tapas Fleming and derived from yoga and Chinese medicine. The TAT is known for its gentle calming effect on distress related to trauma. This technique has also been used successfully with allergies to food and other substances in the environment.

The TAT "pose" involves touching the tip of the thumb just above the inside of one eye and the tip of the ring finger just above the inside of the other eye so that these two fingers are on either side of the bridge of the nose. Place the tips of the index and middle fingers on the "third eye" point just above and between the two eyebrows. Place your other hand across the occiput (the bony ridge across the middle of the back of your head).

It may be a good idea to read through the steps of the protocol below before you start. You will be holding the TAT pose for a few minutes, so please make sure your arms are supported in the pose. A pillow can be folded and placed under the elbow of the arm that

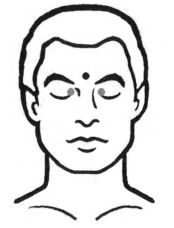
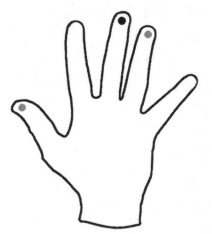

The TAT

is holding the points, and you can lean back against a pillow or the back of a comfortable chair to support the arm that is holding the back of the head. It is certainly OK to take breaks between the steps to stretch and shake out any tension. DO NOT allow your body to be in pain with this pose—it's important to modify it in any way that makes sense to you. If necessary, drop the holding of the back of the head (occiput) and focus only on the points around the eyes and on the forehead.

Holding the pose described above, complete the following:

1. *Identify the problem. Make sure that the words you choose fully resonate for you. For example, specify that you want to correct energy depletion after talking with family members on the phone, or emotional and physical distress after meeting with your supervisor at work, etc. The problem, in this case, may be one that seems to accompany a rise or "spike" in your pain levels.*

2. *Do the three boosters: Drink water, do the overenergy correction, and correct for reversals by saying appropriate affirmations out loud and stimulating the sore spot on your left chest, or on both sides (see above).*

3. *TAT Clearing: Hold the pose and think of the pain trigger you want to resolve:*

   Step 1: Think of the problem trigger in your own words—for example, "I feel exhausted after talking with family members on the phone" or "I feel very upset and scared and my pain increases after meeting with my supervisor at work," etc.

   Notice what you feel in your body and the reactions of your mind.

   *Step 2: Put your full attention on the condition that is the **opposite** of the problem trigger in step one. Notice what happens as you hold the TAT pose and breathe.*

   Step 3: Put your attention on the phrase: "All of the origins or root causes of this problem are healing now." Say it out loud while holding the pose. Notice what happens.

Step 4: Holding the TAT pose, put your attention on the phrase, "All the places in my mind, body, and life where this has been a problem are healing now." Repeat this three times and notice what happens.

Step 5: Do the TAT pose and put your attention on the phrase, "All of the parts of me that have ever gotten something out of having this problem are healing now." Repeat out loud three times. What do you notice?

Step 6: Do the TAT pose and put your attention on the following phrase: "I ask forgiveness of everyone I have ever hurt because of this problem." Say it out loud three times. What happens?[10]

Step 7: Holding the TAT pose, put your attention on the phrase, "I forgive everyone I have ever blamed for this problem, including God and myself." Say this phrase out loud several times. Notice what happens.

*End the pose, stretch, and shake out your arms. Then go back to the problem statement related to your pain trigger. Do you react differently now to this phrase? How? You can repeat the exercise with the same trigger as many times as you wish and use TAT with **any** problem related to pain.*[11]

Exercise: **The Eight-Point Protocol for Emotional or Physical Pain and Related Stress**

Numerous Energy Psychology and Energy Medicine methods are effective with physical and emotional pain. The protocol below is very flexible and can be used with any type of physical pain, with any negative beliefs or painful emotions connected with pain, and with any elements of experience related to pain, including traumatic events. It is modified from the EFT (Emotional Freedom Technique), an Energy Psychology technique developed by Gary Craig.[12]

EFT and its precursor, Thought Field Therapy or TFT, developed by Dr. Roger Callahan, are called **meridian** therapies. That is, they work by stimulating points along the twelve major (and other minor) energy meridians or pathways in the body. The basic structure for EFT and TFT is called a *sandwich* since the protocol is to stimulate eight acupuncture points (or acupoints) followed by a brain-balancing sequence designed to balance left/right brain functions (considered to be the "filling" of the sandwich), and then to restimulate the same eight acupoints. Read through the protocol first before working your way through it.

The eight-point protocol is relatively easy to learn and can be used with virtually any issue related to pain. For example, you can learn to apply this protocol to fears related to pain, to the experience of pain itself, and to the stress and exhaustion pain can cause. Here are the steps:

1. First, identify the problem—for example, fear of an increase in your pain, and rate its strength. Allow yourself to feel the fear (or other problem) as strongly as possible. Give your experience of the problem a number from 1 to 10 (with 10 being as strong as it has ever been) in terms of how strong the problem you want to treat feels right now at the present moment. This number will give you a baseline in order to measure the change that takes place.

2. Complete the three boosters (see above) as they relate to this problem. Drink at least a full 8-ounce glass of water, rebalance the energy system by doing the overenergy correction, and create a positive energy field by correcting for energy reversals using the affirmations.

3. Next, choose a reminder phrase connected to the problem you want to work with (see step 1). Its purpose is to help you stay tuned into the problem throughout the energy treatment. For our example, it might be "fear that my pain will increase" or even just "my fear." Make sure you resonate with the words as fully as possible, so try out different phrases and check your body's biofeedback to make sure you feel fully connected to the phrase you choose. Repeat the phrase out loud as you stimulate each of the following points identified in #4.

4. Now stimulate the eight acupoints by tapping or rubbing gently on each point, or by touching the point and breathing. If you are in severe pain, I recommend that you start with gently touching the prescribed point with one finger, holding the point lightly, and then take a slow, deep breath in and out before moving on to the next acupoint. **Say out loud the reminder phrase** as you stimulate the following points on either side of the body or both sides. Check the diagrams below to find each point before you begin:

A good rhythm with this is to **stimulate the point while saying out loud** "fear about my pain increasing" or whatever your reminder phrase is. Take at least one deep breath in and out and move on to the next point until you have stimulated all eight points.

The protocol would go something like this:

"My fear" 1 - Eyebrow point near bridge of nose—Breathe

"My fear" 2 - Side of eye on the bone bordering on the edge of the eyebrow—Breathe

"My fear" 3 - Under the eye on the bony ridge there—Breathe

"My fear" 4 - Under the nose—Breathe

"My fear" 5 - Under the lower lip—Breathe

"My fear" 6 - The collarbone points—Breathe

(From the tiny notch on the collarbone on either side of the midline of the body, come down one inch and over one inch toward the shoulder.)

"My fear" 7 - Under the arm points—four inches below armpit—Breathe

"My fear" 8 - "Karate chop" or side of the hand points—Breathe

5. When you have finished the eight points, check back in with the problem you started with and give it a new number of intensity or distress. If you are making progress, change the reminder phrase and restimulate the eight points again. For example, if your fear about your pain increasing now seems less, you might want to treat whatever is left of the fear. Change your reminder phrase to "What's left of this fear" and

*repeat the eight-point protocol above. If you are not making progress,
you may want to check for and clear other reversals, try the "sandwich approach"[13], or add the additional points below not included in
the 8 point protocol.*

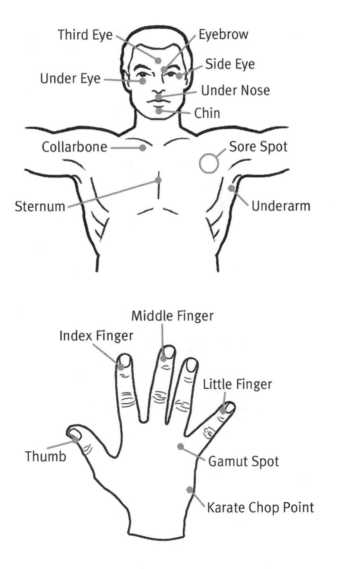

Major Tapping Points

How far down did your fear level (or the level of the particular problem you chose) go this time? Repeat again until you get as close to zero as you want to go.

You can repeat this exercise as often as you like with any problems you encounter during the week, even if they don't seem to be connected to your pain condition. Over time you will develop more confidence in this rapid method for regulating your pain.

Combining Energy Psychology with Other Methods

One of the most exciting avenues of growth in the Energy Psychology field involves adding EP techniques to the EMDR (Eye Movement Desensitization and Reprocessing) model.[14] EMDR is one of the newer methods used to treat trauma, and research has indicated very promising results in healing many types of post-traumatic problems. Although the exact ways that EMDR creates change are unknown, the theory is that it helps restore the mind-body information processing system that has been disrupted by trauma.

Therapists who are trained in EMDR ask clients to focus on some aspect of a traumatic event (which might include images, body sensations, emotional feelings, or related thoughts and beliefs), in order to turn on the individual's informational processing system. Next, the therapist uses some form of bilateral stimulation to activate alternating eye movements, or alternating sensory experiences through tapping or audio sounds, which is believed to stimulate accelerated information processing that unlocks disturbing information that has blocked memory networks and moves it toward a state of balance and integration.

Although EMDR has been recognized for its effectiveness in helping a traumatized person rapidly reprocess multiple dimensions of traumatic memories, caution is urged with self-practice of EMDR outside of sessions with trained professionals. For this reason, I have not included EMDR as a self-treatment method with chronic pain. However, when bilateral stimulation is combined with several EP methods, there is greater safety for self-use, while maintaining the speed and effectiveness of EMDR reprocessing.

Exercise: **The Butterfly Hug**[15]

This technique was created by professionals in Mexico to help children involved in natural disasters. The children are asked to hug themselves and then tap their shoulders gently in alternating rhythm, thus mimicking the movement of butterfly wings.

To use the butterfly hug, think of a time recently when your pain experience was surprisingly easier in some way. As you think of this time, cross your arms over your chest so that your hands are touching either shoulder. While still thinking of this time of "easier pain," tap your shoulders very gently in an alternating rhythm, first one and then the other. Continue for several minutes. This is a way of "sealing in" this positive experience and combines the bilateral stimulation of EMDR with the tapping of neurolymphatic ("sore spot") points near the shoulders.

What is this like for you? This approach can also be used to help you through a time when you are triggered and your pain unexpectedly increases. Try the "butterfly hug" the next time you are surprised by a pain spike. What happens? You may also feel free to teach this to others, including children, as it has been proven consistently to be a safe and positive method.

Exercise: **WHEE**

Another "hybrid" of EMDR and EP is the WHEE (Whole Healing Easily and Effectively) method.[16] WHEE involves three simple steps and is equally effective with complex problems such as chronic emotional and physical stress and pain, as well as more one-dimensional ones.

To use WHEE, use the 3 boosters and then:

1. *Identify a feeling or thought you would like to change. The more specific you can be, the more likely you will be to get resolution. Examples are: "I want to resolve this stabbing pain in my back" or "I want to resolve this throbbing pain in my hip (or neck, leg, side, foot, etc.)." Give it a number of intensity on a scale from 0 (not distressing) to 10 (the most distressing it could be). Children who don't know numbers yet can hold their hands apart a distance to show how big the "bad" feeling is.*

2. *Alternate stimulation of the right and left side of the body in some way. This can be done by alternately tapping the right and left eyebrow points at the ends nearest the nose, by tapping the right and left shoulders in the butterfly hug (see above), by moving the eyes right to left and left to right, or any other kind of alternating tapping method.*

3. *While tapping, recite an affirmation: "Even though I have this stabbing pain in my back and I'm angry that it's not gone, I deeply and completely love and accept myself and my body" or "Even though I have this throbbing pain in the right side of my neck and I'm afraid I can't get rid of it, I deeply and completely love and accept myself." If it fits for you, you can add the phrase "and God loves and accept me wholly and completely and unconditionally," following the self-affirmation.*

After tapping for a few minutes, check the pain number again, and change the target and affirmation to reflect any changes. (Example: "Even though I still have *some* of this stabbing pain in my back, I fully accept myself and my body.") Continue tapping.

If the numbers don't decrease, massage the thymus point located just below the collarbone in the middle of the sternum, which also corresponds to the heart energy station or chakra, without using an affirmation. Diaphragmatic breathing (or another favorite breathing technique) can help deepen these results. Then repeat the three steps above.

If you are worried about tapping in public, you can tap with your tongue on the left and right teeth or even imagine yourself tapping your body to get similar results.

SUMMARY: So far in this chapter, you learned three benefits about lasting relief and how Energy Psychology and Energy Medicine approaches can help you align yourself with what is true about permanent relief. You practiced three ways to "boost" the effects of any energy treatment, and read how drinking water can help you get your energy moving, how the overenergy correction can help rebalance your energy system, and how you can create a positive energy field by correcting reversals through affirmations and acupoint stimulation. You also had a chance to experiment with the TAT in relation to pain triggers and with the eight-point energy protocol to clear aspects of your emotional or physical pain. Next you will learn the wisdom of a regular practice of energizing yourself to start each day in a positive direction.

Body Awareness Skill #6

ENERGIZE Yourself to Maximize Your Pain Relief

Use Energy Psychology techniques to start your morning off with positive energy. This sequence of three short techniques is designed to treat the traumatizing aspects of your pain condition. Create a 2- to 5-minute energy practice that you can do every morning to balance your energy system and interrupt your trauma responses related to pain. If you do this consistently, you will find that you start the day with more energy and more confidence about managing your pain. You'll recognize that two of the three energy techniques are also two of the three "boosters."

1. The Three Thumps.[17] *You may want to start with this simple exercise to turn on positive energy, boost the immune system, promote mental clarity, and strengthen vitality. There is some evidence to suggest that the Three Thumps also help to interrupt the freeze or dissociation response.*

"Thump" or rub the K-27 points just under your collarbone. As in the eight-point protocol (above), these points are located one inch below and one inch out toward the arm from the small collarbone notch near the body's midline. NOTE: These are not the same as the sore spot on your chest near your shoulder crease.

"Thump" or stimulate the thymus point, which is in the middle of your sternum or chest. You should actually hear a "thump."

"Thump" or rub (much easier) the spleen points, which are just under your breasts in line with the nipples.

How do you feel as a result of the Three Thumps?

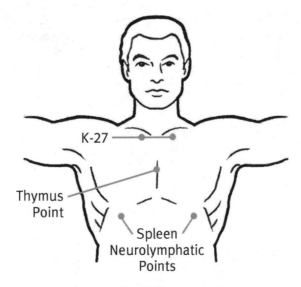

The 3 Thumps

2. Overenergy Correction. *You might want to add this in next for calming and centering, and for countering panic, anxiety, and worry. As you know, too much stress or trauma activation can disorganize your energy flow. See the steps on pages 109–110, above.*

3. Affirmations. *Create a positive energy field to start the day. Rub the "sore" spot on your left chest (this is not the K-27 or collarbone point but the spot closer to the arm crease—see page 119 above) and say some affirmations out loud that are appropriate for how you are feeling and what you anticipate the day will be like. (Example: "I deeply and completely love and accept myself even though I have more pain this morning . . . or even though I dread what I have to do today. . . ," etc.)*

You can then add any other practice such as mindfullness meditation or conflict-free imagery. Also consider the TAT if you are aware of a pain trigger, or the eight-point protocol if you'd like to work with other aspects of your pain.

Use your intuition to sequence these energizers. Try these methods for a week or until you feel confident with the results you get. Attempt to make this a regular morning practice, or use at some other time (or several times) during the day. It is also helpful to use energy approaches in the late afternoon when your energies are usually lower.

CHAPTER SEVEN

Move
Make the Right Moves for Your Body

Every notable reference on chronic pain emphasizes the importance of **exercise.** There are several key benefits of regular exercise for people in pain: 1) Exercise boosts endorphins, which are brain chemicals that create feelings of well-being in the body; 2) Exercise increases the brain's output of serotonin to boost mood; 3) Levels of norepinephrine are increased through regular exercise, which also enhances mood and energy; 4) Exercise helps stabilize estrogen for women; 5) Exercise improves overall brain functioning—brain imaging shows that exercise "lights up" the brain with increased physical energy.

Yet, if you are like many chronic pain patients, you have experienced episodes of feeling more pain when exercising and perhaps even endured significant setbacks due to overuse or misuse of body parts during exercise. Even more frustrating, you may have experienced the confusion of receiving contradictory messages about exercise from professionals who treat pain conditions, such as "use it or lose it," "go slow so you don't re-injure yourself," or "expect some soreness but stop if there is pain." How does one translate this kind of conflicting advice into an exercise program that really works? Hannah's story is a good example of this challenge.

⌣ HANNAH

Hannah, a client with patellofemoral syndrome (dysfunction of the kneecap and knee joint), was referred by her physical therapist (PT) to a fitness center for swimming, aquatics exercise classes, and work with the leg press machines. Her PT had helped her construct a workout program of about 45 minutes and supervised her in work with the leg press to make sure she had the correct settings and was attempting an appropriate number of repetitions.

When Hannah joined the gym, she made an appointment for a fitness instructor to start her on the equipment, a requirement for all new members. Michael, her enthusiastic instructor, was very knowledgeable and encouraged her to test her limits: "I lost 150 pounds in nine months because I kept at it, even when I didn't want to. It will be a struggle at first, but if you just do a little bit more than you think you can each time you exercise, you will achieve your goals."

Fortunately, Hannah was self-confident enough to follow her own body's feedback. She stopped *before* she felt pain, using distress signals from her knee to stop an exercise sequence when she felt soreness even though Michael was encouraging her to "breathe through it." Later, when they talked about her experience, Hannah asked Michael if he had ever had a pain condition. When he admitted that he had not, Hannah commented, "If you'd ever been in pain for a while, you would want to avoid going there again any way you could. For some people, soreness might be a good thing. I've learned that for me, it's a warning signal that I need to respect."

Hannah's experience raises some common questions. How much exercise is enough? How much is too much? When do you push through pain? When do you back off? What kind of exercise is best and how do you use your body's feedback to chart an effective program?

Solving the Puzzle of Exercise: Rediscover Your Body's Design

Pete Egoscue is a well-known physical therapist who has designed an approach to exercise for pain patients known as the Egoscue method. He points out that when pain warns us of danger, we often misinterpret the danger message by being overly careful of making "the wrong move." Unfortunately, what can happen is that we stop making the right moves or any moves at all.

According to Egoscue, the real danger is "motion starvation." That is, if we respond to our body's "danger" signals by guarding or constricting our muscles to protect ourselves from further injury and pain, we run the risk of *not moving enough* to work our muscles in the ways they were designed to move, so that eventually they become too weak to do their job.

The 3 R's of Egoscue's program are: 1) Rediscover the body's design, 2) Restore the body's natural function, 3) Return to health. His major principle is that the muscles, tissues, bones, nerves, and joints will only retain their functions through regular use. Like scaffolding built to support a certain amount of weight, the body is designed to be used for certain supportive functions. If it is not used in alignment with designed functions, much like scaffolding, the body will sag or collapse.

Muscles that forfeit their full range of motion gradually lose their design memory. Peripheral muscles will take over some of this lost functioning, but gradually their design function is compromised as well, forcing the body to search further. Although the body is extremely resourceful and will find unique combinations of compensatory muscles, gradually these too will lose their own design memory and become compromised as well. Less and less able to move, the body's muscles will depart even further from their designed way of functioning. The resulting immobility causes all of the muscle groups to continue to lose their design memory, which renders them less and less able to move, contributing to a vicious circle of further immobility.

Egoscue uses the principle of bilaterality to diagnose areas of the body that have lost their design memory.[1] Because each side of the body is designed as a mirror image of the other, the right shoulder is compromised if it does not look and act identically to the left shoulder, and the left hip to the right, the right arm to the left arm, and so forth. When both sides of the body do not operate in an identical manner, the whole musculoskeletal system begins to be misaligned.

Exercise: Take a Motion Break instead of a Coffee or Tea Break

*Keep a **motion diary** in your pain notebook for a few days to find out which parts of the body are getting too little activity compared to others that may be overused. Are you surprised by your findings? Expand your patterns of motion by adding one non-patterned movement per hour. For example, if you are sitting for most of your workday, stand up to break the pattern. If you are mostly reaching in front of you, reach behind you or above your head. Other examples include looking up at the ceiling, moving your head as far as possible to the right and then to the left, kneeling, standing on a chair, and rolling on the floor. Try one pattern-breaking movement every hour for one 6- to 8-hour period. What do you discover?*

Prepare for and Recover from Exercise

Getting Started. If you are just returning to exercise after an injury, or if you have not exercised regularly for some time for other reasons, please consult a professional to design a program specifically for your needs *and* to supervise you to make sure the program is a good fit for you. Some types of professionals that would be appropriate to consult are physical therapists, physiatrists, Pilates instructors, yoga instructors, and personal trainers with experience in working with chronic pain patients. If you are in doubt, ask your treating professionals for referrals. It is best to plan to work with a trained professional during the first part of your return to exercise.

The fear of experiencing pain from exercise can be a major barrier to resolving any chronic pain condition. Remember that it will take a while to settle into an exercise routine that creates positive benefits, such as strengthening and reconditioning your body. *This is because your body and mind need to be trained to work together effectively* in the context of stretching or exercise. You may be "out of practice" at this or you may never have gotten into the practice of mind-body partnership before now.

So what takes a long time is *not* learning the steps of the exercise program, or how to prepare and recover from it, but how to help your thinking mind and your feeling body come into alignment. This process is something like helping two people who speak different languages communicate with each other. And this sometimes takes more time and effort than we would like.

One of the first challenges is identifying the sensation of soreness related to the fatigue of exercising muscles unused to a workout. This is not the same as your chronic pain, but if you are scared or anxious, the sensations can feel very similar. If you plan to exercise regularly, you need to expect delayed muscle soreness. This is a positive sign that your body is building new muscle and tissue. This type of delayed soreness usually occurs the day after or even longer following your workout. If you experience pain in the injured area immediately or several hours after your workout, more than likely this is a sign that you are pushing too hard and that you need to ease into exercise more slowly and gradually.

If you have a pain flare-up from exercise, always talk to your fitness consultant to decide whether eliminating certain activities, doing fewer repetitions, or other modifications would be best for you. *The cardinal rule here is: Always err on the side of caution. Less is more.* That is, if you are uncertain how to modify your exercise program so that you can avoid reinjury or pain elevations, be more conservative rather than pushing yourself. This is not a case of "getting back on the horse" so that you won't be afraid to exercise. This is a case of being a good steward of your body's vulnerability so that you are able to continue exercising on a regular basis.

Warming Up

There is minor controversy as to whether pain patients should stretch before they warm up, and there are good arguments both ways. A "middle of the road" approach is to warm up for 3–5 minutes by walking while swinging your arms just to get your blood flowing, or by doing the activity you are about to do during your exercise workout but at a much lower intensity (slower and without any strain). Then you can move into stretching.

Stretching

Stretching is one of the best ways of improving your body's flexibility. It is also important before and after aerobic exercise to release constriction and prevent stiffness. Certain types of stretches may even relieve some kinds of pain related to cramped or too-tight muscles.

The benefits of stretching include the following:[2]
- Helps the body relax and feel good
- Allows easier and freer movement
- Increases range of motion
- Helps prevent injury
- Prepares your body for activity

- Maintains and expands flexibility
- Helps develop body awareness
- Helps loosen the mind's control of the body so that the body moves for the sake of moving

Stretching can be done at different times: in the morning to ease into the day, at work to release stress and stiffness, after sitting, standing, or holding one position for a long period of time, when you feel stiff or sore, or any time during another activity throughout the day or evening when you think about it.

Bob Anderson, an expert on stretching, emphasizes that you cannot hurt yourself by stretching *unless* you are rushing or in a hurry to "get it over with" and your body is not relaxed, *or* you push too far (for example, overstretching a cold or previously sore muscle), *or* you fail to pay attention to how the stretch feels in your body.

Always stop if you are uncomfortable, even if you believe you "should" be able to do the stretches easily. This is not a contest to prove you can do it. And it is best to avoid stretching a recently injured or inflamed muscle and its surrounding tissue. If in doubt, do not stretch!

If you have been given a set of stretches to do by a trained professional but have discontinued them because of time constraints, or because they did not seem to help you significantly, retrieve them from your memory banks. If you truly cannot remember the steps you were asked to go through when stretching, it might be worth a call or email to the physical therapist or other professional who gave you the stretches to make sure that you are doing them correctly. The recovery of many pain patients gets derailed because they either don't do the stretches over a long enough period of time, or because they are doing the stretch incorrectly.

If you have not been given stretches to do for your pain condition, try one or both of the general stretches below. [Please note that these stretches are not designed to take the place of consultation with a trained expert.]

1. Do a simple calf stretch. Cross your forearms and lean them on a wall. Rest your forehead on the back of your hands. Bend one knee and bring it toward the wall. Keep the back leg straight with the foot flat and pointed straight ahead, or slightly turned in if pointing the back foot straight ahead is uncomfortable. Hold a very easy stretch through your back calf for about 5–10 seconds. Do not strain and do not bounce. Now reverse legs to stretch the other calf.

2. Lie on your back with your arms stretched overhead. Slowly straighten both legs but do not lock your knees! Point your toes away from your body. Feel a gentle stretch through your arms, shoulders, spine, abs, as well as rib cage, ankles, and feet. This is a stretch that can be done while lying comfortably in bed.

Do your stretches in an *easy* manner. Pretend you are moving in slow motion. Below are tips to avoid problems with stretching:

- DO NOT bounce your body when you go into a stretch. Stretch only to the point where you feel a mild tension that is comfortable for you. Breathe into the stretch and make sure your body is relaxed. When you are bending or moving your body, exhale while bending or moving and then breathe slowly and easily while you hold the stretch for 5–10 seconds.

- DO NOT hold your breath while you stretch. If the tension of the stretch increases while you hold it, ease off slightly until the tension is comfortable again. It may help you at first to count the seconds while you are holding the stretch as a way of keeping your mind focused and aiming for the recommended amount of time.

- DO NOT cause pain. When you push too far, the body will constrict or tighten to protect itself, and you will end up tightening the muscles you want to stretch and loosen. Stretching too far or too fast may result in tearing the muscle fibers at a microscopic level, which ends up making the muscles stiff and sore.

Your goal with stretching is to enjoy the feeling and to look forward to the experience of loosening or flexibility. If this is not happening, stop and reread the directions. Then modify your approach until you experience enjoyment and relaxation. When you achieve this, your mind and body will be working together in a truly effective partnership!

Success with Your Exercise Program

If you are in a lot of pain or significantly deconditioned, it may be best to start with gentle exercise activities. These may include warm water walking, brisk walking outdoors or on an indoor track, tai chi, Pilates mat exercises, swimming, cycling, and yoga. All of these provide good benefits and do not place excessive strain on joints or major muscles.

Whatever exercise you choose, start with five minutes or whatever duration you can complete without hurting during or afterward. If you end up feeling like you don't want to exercise again any time soon, you've done too much. If you feel frustrated because you are not getting "good enough" results, work on your attitude toward yourself. Use the affirmation approach you learned in Chapter Six to correct reversals. (For example: Say aloud, "I deeply and completely love and accept myself even though I am frustrated by having to go so slowly with exercise" while stimulating the point one inch down from your collarbone on the left side of your chest and three inches toward your left shoulder; or use the eight-point protocol to clear your frustration or anger.)

REMEMBER: If you end your exercise period wanting more, that's good because you will be more likely to come back for more.

In addition, the following guidelines can help you be more successful with your exercise program:

1. Schedule exercise as a regular part of your day. Do not wait until you feel "ready" to exercise. Plan it just as you would any other type of treatment.

2. Increase your commitment by involving other people. Take a walk or go to an exercise class with a friend. Find an exercise buddy.

3. Enroll in a class designed for people with injuries. This can include special yoga classes, water aerobics and water walking classes, and spin classes.

4. Plan your exercise at a time of day when you can be successful. If you are not a morning person, don't expect yourself to roll out of bed to be the first person at the gym or pool. If you hate driving in rush-hour traffic, don't expect yourself to take a class scheduled just after the workday. If you are exhausted in the late afternoon and need to nap or rest, schedule exercise before or after those times.

5. Sometimes it can be worth the money to hire a personal trainer. He or she can tailor an exercise program uniquely for you, and you are more likely to show up if you must pay for any regular sessions that you miss.

Cooling Down

Toward the end of your exercise period, continue the same type of exercise you were doing, gradually going more slowly until your heart and respiration are at a resting rate. Then stretch again as you did above to prevent muscle stiffness or soreness.

Recovering Afterward

If you feel delayed muscle soreness hours after exercising, take a warm bath, apply heat to affected muscles, always apply ice if there is swelling or inflammation and/or massage the muscle yourself or get a professional to do so for you. You can do all of the above immediately after exercising to prevent delayed soreness. You may also take an over-the-counter anti-inflammatory after the soreness begins. It is important not to take this medication as prevention *before* you exercise, however. This is because doing so might hide physical reactions that are important for you to be aware of.

Hot and Cold Therapies

When doing exercises or stretching programs, don't forget about the simple use of heat and ice!

Cold is the best choice for acute injuries such as a pulled muscle and for pain flare-ups related to exercise. Cold constricts the blood flow to painful areas of the body and relieves inflammation. It also reduces the flow of pain-causing chemicals such as lactic acid, relieves muscle spasms, and stimulates endorphin release.

Cold is usually applied in the form of ice bags, cold packs, or even by applying bags of frozen vegetables! Cold is commonly used for pain related to arthritis, bursitis, muscle pain, and migraines to numb affected nerves. Caution: Cold treatments should not be used more than 10–15 minutes per session.

Heat is particularly helpful in relaxing muscles and is commonly used for arthritis, back pain, muscle spasms, and fibromyalgia to increase blood flow and flexibility. Heat is usually applied with hot packs, heating pads, and hot baths. Microwavable heat packs are especially convenient. Heat is also useful for softening muscles before or after massage.

Ultrasound is used to heat connective tissue through high-frequency waves. Unlike other forms of heat therapy, ultrasound waves penetrate the outer layer of muscle so that it can heat the inner structures of muscles and connective tissues. This treatment works best for acute injuries and for sprains and strains.

Caution: Do not use heat on actively inflamed joints. Do not use heat if you have neuropathy, diabetes, Raynaud's disease, or any other condition that prevents you from feeling temperatures normally. Heat treatments should be used for no longer than 10–15 minutes at a time.

Many pain therapists recommend *alternating* heat and cold during the same session. For some types of pain, this may be more effective than either alone. To find out what is best for you, consult your treating professional.

Cope with the Challenges of Exercise with Healing Touch

One of the oldest forms of healing techniques for pain is **touch.** When medical professionals had more time, they could use their hands to soothe, comfort, probe, or explore. There is research to show that doctors who touch patients in the hospital on the shoulder or hand, or who sit on their beds, tend to have patients who recover more rapidly with less pain.

Because today's doctors and nurses have such tight schedules, they may not take time to touch. This is especially unfortunate because many pain patients are touch-deprived, partially because the pain itself discourages touch by others, but also because depression, anxiety, and irritability related to pain can build a wall that keeps others at a distance. However, touch deprivation can also intensify the hurt.

Massage

This is one of the most universally effective forms of healing touch for chronic pain. In addition to providing comfort and all-over feelings of well-being, massage has the benefits of loosening tight muscles and improving circulation. Massage has also been shown to work directly on the nervous system, reducing "substance P," a neurotransmitter that helps communicate pain signals throughout the body, and increasing "feel-good" endorphins. Research also indicates that massage helps to reduce cortisol, a stress-related chemical, and to improve sleep.

Because massage is so valuable, if you can afford weekly or bimonthly sessions, it is best to schedule treatments regularly, since the positive effects are cumulative and build over time. As an alternative, you might want to reserve massage for a pain flare-up, for breakthrough pain that does not respond to usual medications or other tools, or when you anticipate a time-limited intense period of stress. As an alternative, ask a loved one to give you a massage. Even though untrained, friends or family members can learn to touch you in ways that bring relief and comfort. Another idea is to take a massage course with a friend or partner and exchange massages on a regular basis.

Though there are many effective types of massage, one of the most common methods is *Swedish massage*, which is designed to relax muscles and improve circulation. Swedish massage is believed to be effective with fibromyalgia. *Deep tissue massage* and *myofascial release* are effective with deep tissue pain and can release the fascia tissue that surrounds bones, nerves, and other internal structures. *Trigger point massage* is useful to disrupt knots of muscles that are tender when pressed and can cause pain to radiate outward through surrounding muscles and tissues. *Sport massage* can break up scar tissue related to injury and help rebalance the muscle system. *Craniosacral massage* is practiced by osteopaths, chiropractors, and some massage therapists to manipulate the soft tissue and sutures of the skull where the bony plates meet. This technique also regulates the energy that pulses from the skull down the spine to the sacrum. Individuals who suffer from headaches and/or jaw or face pain can be particularly helped by this approach, as well as those whose history includes significant past trauma.

Whatever type of massage you prefer, please make sure that your practitioner has been professionally trained and has the proper licensure or certification. Also make sure that the person is comfortable for you to be with and is someone you can trust. It is *essential* that you give your body practitioner information about your medical problems, especially sensitive or reactive areas in the body, and your preferences for types of touch. You will also need to speak up during massage sessions to direct or correct your practitioner's methods. A skilled, trusted massage therapist can be a great ally in helping you move through any discomfort or pain and in encouraging increased body awareness and pleasurable feelings.

Caution: Do not use massage if you have a tumor, cancerous growth, or systemic infection such as lupus or shingles, as massage can cause this to spread. Consult your physician if in doubt.

Exercise: **Self-Massage**

Many pain patients have never given themselves a massage, believing they don't know enough or that their touch is not as "good" as that of a professional and will therefore not be effective.

a. Get out your favorite lotion or oil, put on relaxing music, and begin to massage the particular area of your body that is sensitive or in pain. Be mindful of your body's feedback to massage those areas that may feel neglected or need special attention at this particular time. [As a challenge, you might want to try **using your non-dominant hand,** *as this can give you a more free, spontaneous touch.] Use soft, slow, exploratory movements. Your goal is not to apply intense pressure but to bring parts of your body comfort and pleasure. Once you start the massage of a particular body area, do not lift your hand off your body for a full five minutes. The idea is to deepen the touch you use so that you stay with it rather than avoiding or hurrying your exploration. As you massage, focus* on the kinesthetic touch your hand is feeling as it massages, as well as the experience of your body as it is massaged. If you want to add a step to practice **pendulation** (see Chapters Two and Three), shift your attention back and forth between your felt sense of the massaged area and the hand that is massaging.

What is this experience like for you? If you'd like, record your impressions here. Try brief self-massage every day for a week. What happens?

b. You may also want to try **trigger point therapy**[3] as a second experience or as an alternative to self-massage as indicated above. Trigger points are highly irritable points, usually found in muscle surrounding the affected area of discomfort. They can be created when a nerve ending at the point becomes hypersensitized due to mechanical, emotional, or chemical stress, or some combination of these. They are not only painful when pressed, but when active they provoke pain or soreness some distance away.

First, find the trigger point by gently searching the area of discomfort into the surrounding muscle. The trigger point will usually feel swollen, sore, achy, or nodular. For best results, breathe in then press gently with a finger or thumb and hold for several seconds while breathing out. If you feel a release or letting go, hold steady while breathing in then press a little deeper while breathing out. If you encounter pain instead of release, back off and find another point in the same general area that is less sore to the touch. Continue this process as needed. As a self-treatment technique, trigger point therapy can be used to provide significant relief in a few minutes for sensitive areas. If the problem persists, however, it is best to get help to treat the underlying cause. Acupuncture, trigger point massage by trained professionals, and other methods can help.

Acupuncture and Acupressure

These are two of the Chinese medicine approaches most frequently used with chronic pain. Thin, sterile needles in the case of acupuncture, or well-trained fingers in the case of acupressure, are used to stimulate particular points. Solid research[4] demonstrates that acupuncture patients have higher levels of natural pain-relieving analgesic chemicals in their spinal cord after receiving treatments. These chemicals (including opioids) act to close the gates on pain signals and elicit feelings of deep relaxation. In addition, acupuncture patients tend to feel more energy, feel more well-rested, and experience a sense of greater balance in their organ systems.

Cautions: Acupuncture is less effective for pain related to damaged nerves. Also, if your immune system is compromised, your practitioner must monitor you carefully.

Electromagnetic Stimulation

Many chiropractors, acupuncturists, and physical therapists use a special unit with electrodes attached to the painful part of the body to send a mild electrical current into the area. The tingling sensation that results from the current moves through the nervous system faster than pain sensations, and also tends to release tight muscles. If this is effective, you might want to inquire about a personal TENS (transcutaneous electrical nerve stimulation) unit that gives you relief for longer periods of time. This type of healing touch often allows pain patients to expand their activity levels without increased pain.

Magnet therapy for pain patients involves attaching special small magnets to various parts of the body to increase blood flow, help balance the electrical forces in the body, and stimulate release of healing chemicals. Studies have shown that magnet therapy can speed up healing and reduce swelling and pain.

Caution: Consult a trained professional such as a chiropractor or acupuncturist about whether these approaches are appropriate for you and for advice about placement and strength of magnets to be used.

SUMMARY: In this chapter, you received some information about the benefits of exercise. You began to understand "motion starvation" as the body's response to fear of pain, and considered how to begin to help the muscles of the body reclaim their design memory. You learned about the importance of breaking the patterns of movement by taking a "motion break" every hour or so. You then reviewed how to prepare for, warm up and stretch, cool down, and recover from exercise. You learned the importance of enjoying stretching and how to avoid pain. You were reminded that there is "no gain *with* pain" when exercising and received some guidelines for making exercise enjoyable. You then reviewed several types of healing touch stimulation and learned to give yourself a mini-massage or to work with trigger points. For this chapter's final exercise, you will learn how to coach yourself through various negative reactions that come up when you move or exercise.

Body Awareness Skill #7

MOVE: Work with Your Inner Coach to Engineer Pain-Free Movement

Use your imagination to create the perfect inner coach to help you through the development of an effective movement/exercise program. What qualities does this coach need to have? Consider patience, determination, sensitivity, compassion, knowledge and skill with chronic pain, as well as any other traits that are important to you. You may want to model your inner coach after an actual coach, teacher, trainer, or mentor you have worked with so that the process feels more real to you.

Spend a few minutes "consulting" with your inner coach each day in an inner dialogue about movement and exercise. It is generally best to do this just before or just after you exercise or stretch. Follow the plan below or create your own and use this approach for at least a week for best results.

Consider asking the following of your inner coach:

- *Opportunities to share general fears and frustrations about exercise and body movement.*
- *Reminders of how to use your breath to center and focus.*
- *Key words for encouragement like "easy," "relax," "you can do it!"*
- *Guidance in a tension-release or other type of relaxation practice before and after you exercise.*
- *Help with one or more specific movements that cause discomfort for you. Ask your coach to guide you through the process of imagining any uncomfortable movements in slow motion and in ways that are pain-free.*
- *Support for negative reactions to exercise, including any negative beliefs or fears you might have.*

How was this approach for you? What was most effective? Can you experience your "coach" as an ally at this point? If not, what needs to change so that you do? Can you imagine consulting your coach in the future? How will you do this and what results do you anticipate?

CHAPTER EIGHT

Pendulate
Heal the Trauma–Pain Connection

We have discussed the connection between unresolved trauma and chronic pain at several points so far (see Chapter Three). During your reading of this chapter, you will have a chance to examine the trauma–pain connection more intensively, in order to learn how stress related to trauma from your past may be significantly affecting your pain condition.

First, let's agree on a definition of **trauma.** The comprehensive perspective on trauma goes beyond childhood abuse or even catastrophic accidents or illnesses. A simple definition of trauma includes any experience that overwhelms your abilities to cope with it. This can include unexpected losses, the impact of natural disasters, abandonment or neglect, consistent lack of emotional support, and the effects of surgeries and medical procedures, as well as various types of childhood abuse.

As many experts have emphasized, it is not the nature or kind of event that creates trauma—it's the impact that the event has on us. Specifically, it is our perception of *any threat to our survival*. It is here that we look to our animal friends to learn from them about our own physiology of trauma and pain.

Explore What Animals Teach Us about Pain and Trauma

If you have a pet, you have probably observed your pet under stress. If you have a cat, you may have watched its response to the threat of a dog or larger animal. If your pet is a dog, you may have observed its reactions to threats from a larger dog, a horse, a bull, or even a coyote, mountain lion, or wildcat, depending on where you live.

Regardless of the identity of predator and prey, when you see an animal under stress, you will have witnessed a universal expression of the fight/ flight/ freeze response. Any animal being threatened will first freeze instinctively while scanning the environment to evaluate the danger. Next, the animal will use its physical abilities to fight back if that is feasible, or will flee the scene if possible, given the circumstances and its capacity for speed. Failing these options, the animal's nervous system will create a continued freezing or immobility response. The possum, for example, can go into such a profound vegetative state that other animals will leave it for dead—which is where the term "playing possum" came from.

In the wilds, this does not pose a problem. If the animal is killed, the powerful chemicals that are released through the immobility response, which include endorphins, adrenaline, and cortisol, will contribute to a relatively painless death, quickly numbing and shutting down body systems. And if the animal survives, it will return to its normal state of equilibrium following an intense period of discharge, which might include trembling, shaking, and a range of behaviors related to fight or flight such as running or attack movements. It appears that these protective motor mechanisms are encoded in the nervous system and must be completed and released before a pre-alarm balance in the nervous system can be restored. Once this chain reaction is finished, however, the animal demonstrates no lasting ill effects from the experience and resumes its normal, everyday life.

Even pets show evidence of participation in these self-regulatory cycles. My dog Casey appears to be traumatized by loud sounds, such as the screeching of buses and loud trucks. When she first hears the sound, she will tense her body and scan the environment for the source of threat. She will attempt to flee the sounds in any way she can. If she cannot move away from them, once they stop, she will lie down and tremble for several minutes, and her legs may also make what appear to be rapid running movements, which may be attempts to complete defensive motor responses that were interrupted by the freeze response.

We human beings also freeze when confronted with a threatening situation. Unlike animals, however, when we freeze and survive the danger, we usually do not shake and tremble to release the fight/flight/freeze energy from our nervous systems. Such behavior is frowned on in our culture. We are expected to "just get over" the stress, especially if we are not physically injured. If we are injured, we are strapped to gurneys where our bodies cannot move. Even well-meaning medical professionals urge us to move around almost immediately—before the anesthesia of surgery trauma has worn off. A common belief is that discharge behavior is cowardly or overly dramatic and therefore to be avoided in order to bypass possible judgments of other people. And, finally, because we are often in a state of helplessness during or following a traumatic event, we tend to shun reactions that may make us feel or appear even more helpless.

↩ SUZANNA

An example of the freezing response can be found in the history of Suzanna, one of my clients, who suffers from fibromyalgia, lupus, and other health symptoms related to multiple childhood traumas. During one of our sessions, Suzanna related an incident that took place when she was about five years old. She was standing outside a house where her family was visiting when a heavy log became dislodged on the hill above her and rolled rapidly downhill toward her. She described how she was frozen, rooted to the spot and unable to move, as the log hurtled in her direction. Unfortunately, none of the adults present intervened to help her. Suzanna suffered severe contusions and nerve damage as a result of the accident, and almost lost her leg. As you might imagine, Suzanna's emotional responses of fear and helplessness persist many years later, though she is learning to better regulate those trauma reactions using some of the techniques presented in this book.

Understand the Nervous System's Role in Pain

Severe constriction or contraction of the musculoskeletal system occurs during the freeze response that if not released can eventually result in, or contribute to, persistent and chronic pain conditions. In addition, the *kindling* reaction of the nervous system to trauma (see Chapter Three for more information) also contributes to a chronic condition of pain in the body.[1]

A human freeze response that is not discharged can result in a prolonged, intense alarm state that creates excitability and hypersensitivity in the neuron pathways connected to the **amygdala,** the major alarm center for emotional and sensory processing. The amygdala sorts pain data that has been relayed through the spinal cord gating system and then routed by the thalamus through the limbic, cerebral cortex, and sensory cortex systems. Resulting patterns related to freezing and to the hyper-alarm state are deeply imprinted as part of the brain's attempts to help us survive threat.

As a protective mechanism for our organisms, the amygdala becomes automatically reactivated in response to post-traumatic memory fragments such as nightmares or flashbacks and even to subtle external cues such as smells, sounds, and images. Each time the amygdala is triggered by reminders of trauma, an alarm state is sounded all over again. If this reaction becomes a self-sustaining feedback loop, the nervous system will be in a state of perpetual hyper-reactivity, which triggers a perpetual reliving of the trauma.

Muscle groups will tense and brace just as they did during the original event, and the use of these same muscles during routine daily activity can then re-trigger the traumatic event, which leads to a vicious cycle of trauma reactivation—rebracing—further reactivation—further rebracing, and so on.

The persistent alarm state signaled by the amygdala and continued through hyperactivity in the nervous system can lead to a buildup of toxins in the muscle fibers, which can result in the chronic stress and myofascial pain reactions found in fibromyalgia, chronic fatigue, irritable bowel syndrome, and other chronic conditions. In her 2004 study of trauma survivors, Belleruth Naparstek[2] points out that a huge percentage of individuals diagnosed with chronic, intractable pain conditions have been found to have histories containing severe trauma. And chronic late-stage post-traumatic stress, which eventually lowers cortisol levels, may also contribute to a variety of autoimmune disorders.

Trauma Reactivation and Dissociation: The Roller Coaster of Pain

Part of the trauma response involves the protective mechanism of **dissociation.** During the freeze response, the body usually feels numb and detached. If an animal is killed in the immobility state, there is some evidence that it feels very little pain or other sensation. When we as humans experience immobility or shock, we also feel very little sensation. If you have been involved in a minor car accident, for example, you may have experienced a sense of disorientation and distancing from the event itself, as if you were engaged in a waking dream. And, unless you are badly hurt, you may not feel any discomfort until the next day or two, when you are more fully connected with your body again.

This is an example of dissociation,[3] or split awareness. We know we have been shaken up or hurt, yet we do not feel the sensation. There is literally a gap between mind awareness and body experience of the incident. People who experience dissociation during traumatic events report experiences like "I left my body" or "I felt like I wasn't really there." Common dissociative symptoms following trauma can include numbing, disconnection from the body, flashbacks, amnesia and partial memory loss, inability to feel emotions and/or the presence of emotions that are inappropriate (either exaggerated, irrational, or nonexistent) given the reality of circumstances.

Dissociation is an involuntary response, so it is one that we cannot control. It is likely that our usually focused minds become numb and unfocused due to chemicals such as endorphins that are released during the freezing response. Dissociation softens the impact of pain and constriction and disconnects us from the fear that accompanies the freezing—dissociation—hyperactivation cycles that are triggered in the nervous system as a response to trauma.

We humans are not only unable to discharge the energy of freezing through the shaking, trembling, perspiring, and other behaviors that our animal friends routinely practice, but the persistent cycling between hyperarousal and dissociation may actually imprint the traumatic event in more primitive and unconscious ways. Such primitive encoding makes it even more difficult for us to intervene in the trauma pathways that are created in our brain and nervous system, and so they persist over time, locked in as rigid feedback loops that are highly self-reinforcing and seemingly impossible to change.

Anxiety and Fear in the Chronic Pain Cycle

The function of fear is to alert us to danger and potential dangers in our environment. In order to understand further the trauma–pain connection, we need to understand how fear operates within post-traumatic stress reactions.

Terror is considered the most extreme form of fear and is central to the experience of any trauma, related to our perceptions that life itself is threatened. After the threat has passed, the terror reduces to anxiety or fear again but can be reawakened by the retriggering of the original traumatic event. Triggers can come in many forms—visual details, sounds, smells, tastes, sensations, body positions, and even thoughts related to dates on the calendar that signal the anniversary of a traumatic event.

What does fear have to do with chronic pain? We have seen that traumatic stress creates a roller coaster in the nervous system. The person confronted with trauma is flooded first with chemical changes related to freezing and the danger alarm sounded by the amygdala. These signals turn on the sympathetic system, which prepares the body for fight and flight. The subsequent "all clear" signal turns off this reaction and turns on the parasympathetic branch of the nervous system, which slows down the accelerated reactions of heartbeat, blood pressure, and respiration and brings the organism back into balance and comfort again.

With chronic traumatic stress, the danger alarm is *always* turned on so that the nervous system is in a perpetual state of hyperactivation and freezing, which creates chronic constriction and eventually chronic pain if not released. Because dissociation is inherent in the freeze response, the chronic pain patient is flooded with inflammation triggered by the constriction of immobility and by the numbing of dissociation. The person struggling with chronic pain has no way to make sense of the alternating patterns of intense "wired" discomfort and deadness in the body, and no way to interrupt these self-perpetuating, unregulated somatic experiences. Michael's story is a good example of this.

◠ MICHAEL

Michael was bewildered when he came to see me. He had had multiple surgeries on his hand and arm since they were crushed when his car flipped over almost two decades ago when he was in his early twenties. "I don't understand why I'm in constant pain, all of a sudden," he said. "After all those surgeries, I never had bad pain until the last one a year ago, when I was forty. And now it doesn't matter what they give me, it doesn't help with the pain. Can you help me make sense of this?"

I took a trauma history and learned that Michael had had several physical injuries when he was a boy, including bad burns caused by an electrical fire when he was six. I speculated that Michael had learned to cope with the pain of these traumas through dissociating from the pain. That is, in order to survive the pain of the severe burns and the horrible anguish of the treatment for the burns which included soaking in baths and peeling away several layers of skin at a time, followed by skin grafts to replace the burned skin (the treatment is often worse than the pain of the burns themselves), Michael learned to turn off the pain, and the mechanism of dissociation helped him do it.

Just before the last surgery, however, Michael began to feel intense fear for the first time. I explained that the activation of that fear response might have reawakened some of his earlier traumatic fears related to the accidents and the burn treatments he had endured. For a long time, he had not felt the fear, thanks to his skill with dissociation. Yet when his body's reactions finally broke through the wall of dissociation he had constructed, he was plunged into "tidal wave" reactions of his nervous system. The terror he felt was so strong and unexpected that his dissociative defense mechanisms were not strong enough to send Michael back into "freezing."

Ultimately, we were able to use many of the tools presented in this book, including pendulation, to help Michael learn how to regulate his physical pain and the emotional pain of fear and helplessness that had long been walled off from his awareness by the dissociation. At the beginning of our work, Michael was so scared and in such intense physical pain that we needed to develop several **conflict-free images,** including one involving scuba diving (a former hobby of his).

Finally Michael was able to focus on his body experience long enough to explore the **felt sense.** We started by finding that he could recall the felt sense of the expanded world under the ocean, where his body could move freely without pain. The scuba diving imagery served to stimulate sensations of expansion in his body that became strong enough to counter his pain and fear. Michael gradually learned that both his fear of pain and the physical pain itself began to shift when he could feel sensations of expansion and "steer" his attention back and forth until his felt body sense became more neutral.

The psychological aspects of fear play a major role in the chronic pain cycle. Many pain clients experience anticipatory anxiety and helplessness without realizing it. If a rehabilitation procedure has been painful previously, or a particular movement or activity has increased pain levels, people with chronic pain will literally "brace" themselves in preparation for these events, which can further increase the constriction in the body and magnify pain. Or they may avoid situations such as treatments with the potential to trigger the traumatic pain response, which may leave them at risk for a poorer recovery.

The key may be to find ways to "shake off" the shock or immobility response related to chronic traumatic stress so that the nervous system can return to balance, and somatic experience become self-regulated once more. There are many promising new somatic methodologies designed to accomplish this goal. One of the most effective is Somatic Experiencing,® developed by Dr. Peter Levine (see Chapter Two for Levine and the felt sense) and discussed after the exercises below. First let's take a few minutes to explore how fear and anxiety may be impacting your current pain experience and learn some simple ways to shift these feelings.

Exercise: **Learn More about Primitive Fears**

Take a few moments to become quiet and settled. Think of your favorite type of small animal. For example, this may be a rabbit, a bird, a squirrel, or even a chicken. As you think of the animal, create any type of sensory image to help imagine that you are this animal. Now . . . imagine that a much larger animal suddenly comes into the scene. Imagine that this animal presents an immediate and **huge** *threat to your survival. How would you respond to this animal? Would you run, try to fight back, "play dead," or some combination of these reactions? Allow these behaviors to unfold as you respond with your imagination. Try to* **feel** *the responses your body would make in that situation as you experience yourself in the role of prey. Let the scene continue until it is resolved in some way. What is the outcome? What happens in your body?*

Now think of your favorite power animal. It could be a special totem you have discovered or an animal that represents strength, agility, and speed, such as the leopard. Imagine yourself in a beautiful safe place in the world of nature that is your home. Get a sense of your surroundings— the light, the colors, the smells. Feel the sense of freedom and safety that is yours as you are "king" or "queen" of your natural kingdom. Imagine running freely, playing, hunting for food. Imagine that you can "step into" the power animal's body that you are imagining. What do you feel in your body now?

Exercise: **Notice Your Fear and Safety Reactions with Pain**

*This exercise is designed to help you become aware of some of the ways that fear influences your experience of pain. To begin, think of a time in your life now when you do not experience much pain. [Hint: This requires you to think of a conflict-free experience.] In fact, pain might be very far away from your thoughts, awareness, and feelings. This will probably be a time when you are fully engaged in an enjoyable or absorbing pastime such as reading a good novel, playing with the children in your life, taking a soothing hot bath or shower, or talking with your favorite friend. Bring this experience into focus as vividly as you can. Again, tune into your body experience. Where do you experience a relative **comfort zone** in your body? Name some of the sensations that you are feeling that are connected with comfort. This may be a good time to practice using the "language of sensation." Examples are: loose, relaxed, limp, light, tingling, heavy, soft.*

Now . . . think of the time in your life when your pain began to become a chronic condition. If there was an accident, injury, or surgery, think of that. If there was another kind of event that you associate with a worsening of your physical pain, think of that.

[NOTE: It is NOT necessary for you to try to recall the details of any traumatic event here. It is only important that you are attuned to or connected with this time in your life. If your experience becomes too intense, please feel free to stop the exercise. Come back to it later if you'd like. It's also fine to let go of this exercise and move on to another one.]

Focus on your body experience as you think about this time in the past. Notice where you feel tightness or constriction. Gently explore the outer edges of these constricted areas. What do you become aware of? Use the language of sensation to describe the body sensations that you link with constriction or tightness. [Examples include: tense, hot, burning, sharp, throbbing, aching, tight.]

*Now . . . return to the conflict-free experience you identified above—
a time when either you feel less pain, or it is not as much in your awareness. How does your body experience begin to change? You might want
to shift or **pendulate** back and forth a few times to find out whether this
helps you create a more solid sense of change in your pain experience. If
this exercise elicits promising results, make a mental or written note to
practice this method at least once a day during the time when your pain
is likely to be higher (for example, after exercise or intense activity, or at
the end of the day when you are tired, etc.). Take a moment to record
your results here or in your pain notebook.*

Interrupt Retraumatizing Cycles of Pain with Somatic Experiencing®

Although these last two exercises can teach you ways to regulate
some of your responses related to fear, the bigger question is, how
can humans "shake off" the effects of shock and immobility so that the
frozen energies of the nervous system can be released and transformed?
How do we begin to "thaw" out from years of freezing and numbing?

Peter Levine, who has degrees in both Medical Biophysics and Psychology, has developed a model known as Somatic Experiencing (SE).[4]
SE features four phases devoted to skill development and trauma resolution involving the body: preparation and building somatic resources;
learning to track specific sensations; discharging activation of the
fight/flight/freeze response; and returning the body to equilibrium.

One of the important contributions of the SE model is its belief
that you do not have to revisit specific traumatic experiences in order
to discover more about "what happened" or to analyze why the event
may have affected you as it did. SE provides a gentle, gradual way of
working with the trauma response in the body—its effect, not its cause.

You have already experienced **pendulation,** which is one of the
most important skills of the SE model. In the next section, you will

learn more about how pendulation can help you "shake off" trauma-related energies that are trapped in the body and re-regulate your nervous system.

Pendulate to Connect Trauma and Healing Energies

In order to understand pendulation, it is important to know something about the subtle energy flow that circulates through the nervous system. Dr. Levine has envisioned that there are two primary vortices of energy—the trauma vortex and the countervortex, or healing vortex. These energies are related to the continual constriction of trauma, and also to expansion that results from experiences unrelated to trauma.

When we are constricted by trauma and its continual recirculation through our body and nervous system, we are often unable to recognize and support the expansion that new experiences and possibilities bring. Practicing the technique of pendulation helps to create a rhythm between constriction and expansion that eventually allows restoration of balance in the nervous system.

Exercise: More Practice with Pendulation

*Identify the sensations in your body connected to constriction at the moment you are reading this. It is likely that your pain condition is linked to this sense of constriction, along with other tensions and tightness in different parts of the body. Let yourself gently explore these constricted energies. Then notice when your attention begins to shift away from the constricted areas and toward areas of expansion in your body. (Have faith and patience. Your attention really **will** naturally shift!) If you are struggling, think of a conflict-free experience (see exercise 2 above).*

Get a sense of the expanded areas in the body. Then use your breath to move intentionally back and forth between expansion and constriction.

As *you breathe in, focus on the expansion; and as you breathe out, focus on the constriction. (If this is awkward, reverse the order and focus on the constriction as you breathe in and the expansion as you breathe out.) Feel your breath naturally shifting back and forth between the sensations like the rhythm of a pendulum. After a few minutes, what do you notice? Have you discovered any benefits of pendulation? What are they?*

For some people with pain conditions, pendulation[5] *is one of the most effective skills they can learn. If you have layers of trauma that start in childhood, and multiple physical traumas or health problems in addition to pain, spend extra time here until you reach a level of mastery. You may want to make further skill with pendulation your goal for this chapter.*

Resolve Inner Conflicts That Block New Somatic Patterns

Another way that the dynamics of trauma can affect us is that we may develop different parts of our personalities to cope with the overwhelming and conflicting aspects of our trauma experience. For example, one part of us may still feel terrified by the traumatic event and relive this fear whenever we are in unpredictable circumstances that remind us of the past event, while the adult part of us wants to move on with life and is very impatient with the fear reactions related to the past. These two parts would obviously be in conflict with each other and could prevent the learning of better ways to feel and cope with fear reactions.

Thus in addition to learning how to shift the constriction and dissociation of the immobility or freezing response, it is also important to explore inner conflicts that may be preventing you from responding optimally to treatment methods or medication. Generally, these conflicts will be related either to the fear/constriction/freezing response or to the numbing/dissociation response or both. For example, you may have a part that is scared that your pain will only get worse, or that there is no hope for recovery. You may have another part that has learned to block out fear by fixating on your surroundings or by daydreaming or "spacing out."

In Chapter Six (when we studied the energy system), we explored some of the common inner conflicts that seem to accompany chronic pain. At that time, you learned how to use **affirmations** to address some of these conflicts, called *reversals*.

One of these affirmations was:

"I deeply and completely love and accept myself even though ... I believe I can't get over or resolve this pain problem."

In this example, the conflict is that at least one part of the self believes that it's impossible to move beyond chronic pain, while another part believes it *is* possible to resolve the chronic pain condition. The belief that it is impossible to recover from pain is probably related to our fear responses.

Another affirmation from Chapter Six was:

"I deeply and completely love and accept myself even though ... I may not feel ready or willing to do what it takes to resolve this pain problem."

This time the conflict seems to be that one part of the self does not feel connected with a readiness or willingness to do what it takes to resolve the pain problem, while another part (or the rest of the personality) may feel very connected to that readiness or willingness. Affirmations are a good way to correct these kinds of inner conflicts because they involve statements of self-acceptance, which are *unifying* to your personality.

Besides the simple affirmation correction you learned in Chapter Six, another important way to resolve these inner conflicts is to **find help** for the parts of the self who are afraid or who are disconnected from important positive motivations. The next exercise will give you a chance to intervene in your inner struggles and help to build a sense of inner cooperation in approaching your pain condition.

Exercise: **Build Internal Cooperation with the Inner Table Technique**

Try the exercise below, reading through it first so that you will be prepared for the steps involved. Choose a conflict to work with that is important yet not overwhelming, until you become comfortable with the process.

1. *First, identify an* **inner conflict** *that you believe might be preventing you from making progress with your pain self-treatment program. Examples include fears that your pain will only get worse as time goes by vs. determination to do whatever it takes to recover from chronic pain; and disconnection from positive feelings about the future vs. confidence that you will find what it takes to be increasingly successful at regulating your pain. State the inner conflict you choose as a fear or as something that is missing (a disconnection from something positive).*

2. *Try to imagine the part of you that seems to be creating the inner conflict (for example, the part that is afraid, the part that can't feel trust or confidence or hope). What do you know about this part of you? What's your guess as to how old she or he might be? What's the piece of your history that helps to explain this part's struggle?*

3. *Now imagine that you can create a very special place inside where all the parts of you can meet together around a table. You might want to imagine a plushly carpeted staircase reaching down inside to the center of your being where there is a meeting room. Be open to whatever surroundings appear to you.[6] Invite the part of you that is creating the conflict into the meeting room, along with all the other parts of you that are willing to help resolve the conflict. Notice who appears and how they arrange themselves around the table.*

Ask the part involved in the negative aspect of the conflict to present his/her case, explaining beliefs and feelings involved. Then ask the
other parts present to make agreements to offer help and support to
this part. You may also want to include your inner coach from the end
of Chapter Seven, if that was a useful experience for you. Make space
for whatever inner dialoguing is needed. End this experience with some
sort of action plan, even if it involves only one small step in the direction of cooperation.

4. End the exercise by recording your experience in your pain notebook or
on a chapter bookmark to remind you to come back for follow-up
"meetings." Track your progress over the next few days. What do you
notice?

SUMMARY: In this chapter, you read more about how pain can be
affected by the roller coaster of traumatic hyperactivation and fear
in the nervous system that alternates with numbing or dissociation.
You also considered how pendulation can gently and slowly begin
to shift this pattern. To examine the role of inner conflicts with
chronic pain, you used the idea of the "inner table" to bring support
and help to the part of you causing the conflict. This chapter's focus
on trauma concludes with a skill that uses some of the techniques
you have learned throughout the book to build new, more expan-
sive experiences in the body.

Body Awareness Skill #8

PENDULATE to Disconnect Pain from Past Trauma

What keeps the roller coaster of pain going in your nervous system
is the connection with past unresolved traumatic experiences, including those connected to the injury, surgery, or illness that triggered
your pain condition, as well as other emotional and physical traumas,

including early childhood trauma. This exercise gives you a way to break that connection.

1. *When you become aware that your body is expressing fear by "bracing" itself, "guarding," or constricting for the next few days (whether or not you are actually **feeling** fear), practice interrupting this pattern by using your favorite type of breathing for a few breath cycles (see Chapter One). When you are actually aware of feeling emotional fear, also practice using your breath to interrupt this response. Remember that it is literally impossible to stay constricted or fearful while you are using the calming breath, foursquare, or the cleansing breath. Try it and see. Are your responses different when using the breath to interrupt physical signs of fear than when interrupting emotional fears? If so, how?*

2. *Think of a time in the last day or two when you felt caught in the trauma activation/ fear/fight/flight response that alternates with the numbing/dissociation/freeze reaction to create the roller coaster in your nervous system. Identify those sensations now in your body (even if they are very minimal) or work with your memory of when they were stronger. Practice pendulation for several moments by shifting your awareness back and forth from tense, constricted, or frozen sensations in your body to sensations or areas of expansion. What happens in your body when you do this?*

3. *If it feels right to do so, bring in your inner coach, trainer, or mentor. Ask for positive feedback regarding what you have learned about the mind-body partnership so far in this book. What information do you receive? Can you take it in without a "yes, but—"? Ask your coach to help identify what is different for you NOW in relation to your pain, when compared with where you were at the beginning of this book. You may also want to ask what your coach believes was missing for you during times of past trauma that is available now in your life— examples include support, human touch, love, compassionate medical help, and so on. Find the felt sense of those possibilities in your body,*

based on here-and-now resources you identify, and pendulate back and forth between these resource areas and remaining areas of constriction, tension, or discomfort.

4. Record your reactions to this exercise in your pain notebook or on a chapter bookmark. Follow up for the next few days, practicing pendulation to continue to disconnect the effects of trauma from your current felt sense of life. Does this help to reduce your pain levels? If you have stopped tracking your daily emotional and physical pain levels (see Chapter Two), please return to this practice now to see how using pendulation to work with signs of past trauma in your body may help to further lower your pain numbers.

CHAPTER NINE

Love
Embrace the Heart of Your Pain

In this chapter you will explore a major contributor to the persistence of physical pain—the emotional pain that can result from unresolved grief and loss or other kinds of emotional shock. I'm sure you already know from your own experience how various types of emotions such as anger, grief, and fear can intensify your pain symptoms.

In Chapter Eight, we reviewed some of the biological evidence that explains how traumatic fear creates constriction in the body that, over time, can lead to a chronic pain condition. You learned that when circumstances are present that evoke a sense of overwhelming threat to our survival, the resulting hyperactivation of the nervous system elicits the freeze/fight/flight response. A cascade of complex chemical reactions as well as muscular constriction creates a persistent alarm state, usually accompanied by (or followed by) a protective numbing or dissociative response. This process creates the complex "roller coaster" that perpetuates the experience of physical pain.

We have not yet examined in any depth, however, the role that grief, anger, and other emotions play in chronic pain conditions. One emotional dimension of pain is the emotional *meaning* you have attributed to your pain. If, for example, your pain was inflicted by another person—such as the drunk driver of the car who hit you, or a doctor's negligence—it is likely that you will experience rage, suffering, and other intense emotional reactions. If, on the other hand, your pain is associated with the relief of surviving or escaping harm, such as getting out of a burning car, it will stimulate a more positive emotional response.

We also know that if more severe injuries are somehow attached to a positive outcome, they trigger less pain and suffering than less severe injuries that might be related to a negative outcome. Researchers have found that soldiers wounded in combat who are to be sent home, for example, experience far less pain than those whose injuries are not as severe but who must remain in the war zone.[1] Therefore, a more positive view of the future and states of positive focus can lessen the emotional suffering of a pain condition. This explains why many athletes are not aware of pain from their injuries while they are absorbed in engaging sports events. Thus mood states associated with positive involvement in a meaningful activity, such as those that accompany the desire to contribute worthwhile achievements to the world or to engage in activities important to the person in pain, are associated with significantly lower pain levels.

Two Peas in a Pod: Emotional and Physical Pain

In order to understand the influence of emotional pain on your physical pain condition, we turn once again to the biology of pain. Unresolved emotional trauma remains active in the nervous system through the dynamics of the limbic–HPA (hypothalamus-pituitary-adrenal) axis. This important regulatory system is balanced by the stress hormone *cortisol.* Under normal conditions, cortisol is released to turn off the sympathetic alarm response and turn on the parasympathetic calming response.

Extreme stress that lasts over a period of months or years, however, severely depletes cortisol levels. This results in disorganized cycling of the HPA axis and the limbic system, the body's emotional center, fluctuating unpredictably between significantly high levels of

cortisol during the high alarm state, and increasing levels of depletion when the alarm lessens. If the limbic center stays in this prolonged alarm state, emotional problems ensue such as depression,
anxiety, anger, fatigue, and fear.

There are several kinds of evidence for how emotional and physical pain are virtually identical from the body's perspective:

1. Physical pain and emotional feelings share common nerve pathways from the periphery of the body to the spinal cord.
2. PET scans of patients with chronic pain show activation of two
   areas of the brain simultaneously, the somatosensory cortex and
   the limbic system. Therefore, incoming pain stimuli activate the
   brain to respond both with painful sensation and emotion.
3. Antidepressants that increase serotonin and norepinephrine
   (chemicals related to depression) relieve both depression and
   physical pain.
4. Previous history with pain affects both current physical and emotional pain experience.
5. Positive emotional factors, such as social and family support, can
   close the gates on both physical and emotional pain.

Crack the Emotional Code of Your Pain and Suffering

Steven Levine, one of the foremost authorities on death and dying,
has turned his more recent attention to the experience of what he
calls "unattended sorrow."[2] Levine claims that we do not know what
to do with our grief and emotional pain. If we try to protect ourselves from pain, we can end up pushing away all that we love, and
feel alone and powerless. Instead, Levine suggests that we must learn
to reenter the parts of ourselves abandoned to the helplessness and
hopelessness of pain, exploring the possibilities of our hearts one
breath at a time.

For most people, sorrow "is the ungrieved losses of love betrayed, of trusts broken, of lies sent and received, of words spoken that can never be betrayed, and of the repeated bruises left by unkindness."[3] Grief related to physical pain includes losing function and mobility. Sometimes pain means there is a job or vocation that we can no longer perform, or the loss of work or marital identity.

Acute grief can be complicated by the loose ends of previous loss. We can often feel that a fresh loss stirs up *all* the losses we have ever had. Because of the enormity of these feelings, during the times when our hearts most need our attention and love, we are least likely to want to give it to ourselves.

Levine believes there are two kinds of chronic grief: the unresolved traumatic grief from earlier losses, and the current grief of disappointments, lost loves, and lost opportunities, all results of life's flow of impermanence that sends our heart's desire in front of us and then moves it away again.

What has broken your heart? As you read this chapter, it is important to consider the unresolved emotional pain that may be affecting the pain you experience in your body. If this feels like an overwhelming task for you, consider working with a trained professional, such as a grief counselor or psychotherapist.[4] Ask yourself, *"What were some of the losses that preceded or occurred around the same time that my pain condition began to be a problem?"* Search for further clues by completing the following exercise.

Exercise: Explore the Language of Pain

Think of some of the adjectives you use to describe your pain. Possibilities are: burning, stabbing, cold, nauseating, shaky, overwhelming, exhausting. Now take each descriptor and consider the question, "What in your life has really 'burned' you? What or who 'stabbed' you in the back or in the heart? What did you find 'chilling'? What has sickened or 'nauseated' you?" And so on.

Make a note of any clues you get about losses or emotional pain that may be connected to the onset of your physical pain condition. This does not mean that any emotional pain or loss you identify **caused** *your physical pain. The point here is that it may not be possible to get* **full** *resolution of your physical pain without treating related emotional pain if there* **is** *an important connection.*

Most people in pain separate from their emotional heartbreak and stay focused on the physical pain. Perhaps it's because pain in the body is more concrete and we have clearer ways of evaluating when we are making progress. Or perhaps because focusing on the emotional heartbreak, in addition to our physical pain conditions, feels much too overwhelming. Yet finding and resolving the source of emotional pain, when sufficient inner strengths have been developed to take on the job, can really help you turn the corner in your pain recovery.

⌐ JENNIFER

Jennifer developed endometriosis like her mother and two older sisters. She followed the recommended treatment, then had several surgeries as her pain intensified. Unfortunately, her work as a commercial photographer required her to stand on her feet for much of the workday and deal with intense work pressure, which amplified her pain significantly. With each surgery, she built up more scar tissue, which eventually triggered more pain, until she found herself in a vicious downward spiral that brought her to my office for help.

After I taught Jennifer some of the same tools you have learned in this book, she began to have less pain on a daily basis, yet negative interactions with her family sent her pain levels back up high again. When we decided to explore the source of her emotional pain, Jennifer revealed that the intensity of her pain had surged to an all-time high jus before her only daughter, Julie, was preparing to leave home after high school graduation. As she told me about some of her struggles with this change in her life, she suddenly clutched her pelvis and said, "This is amazing! My pain level has really shot up just talking about thi ."

Over several sessio s, we gathered more information to pinpoint some of the key even ; that evoked grief and loss related to Julie leaving home and link with Jennifer's own experiences of separating from her alcoholic mily during her high school years. We used imagery and some enei y techniques to release her grief and fears. This emotional work cu her pain levels in half and prepared Jennifer to begin tapering f her medication.

Exercise: **Review the Beginning of Your Emotional Pa**

If you want to go further w the clues you have found so far, you can participate in a structured review of the source of your pain. Read through the following script.[5] If possible, you might want to make an audio recording so that you can listen and respond freely to the exercise. Have your pain journal or notebook ready to record your responses as soon as you finish.

Settle comfortably and quietly. Start with your preferred kind of breathing for a few cycles. Add key words as you breathe in and out, such as "relax" (inhale) . . . "now" (exhale) or "release" (inhale) . . . "tension" (exhale). After a few moments, when you feel comfortable, you can begin the exercise.

A review of emotional heart pain that may be connected to the beginning of your physical pain may give you more control over your symptoms. Each time you review the experience that contributed to your pain condition, or to a time when your pain took a turn for the worse, you will find that you gain more information, and that your current physical and emotional pain will be diminished afterward.

When you are ready, go back to the time just before your pain became worse or became significantly important. What are you doing? Who are you with? Where are you? What happens? What are your emotional impressions? What are you feeling at the moment of the accident, injury, or other event that seems connected to your pain? What is going on for you at the moment your pain became serious or got worse?

Continue your review up to the moment when you know that this experience is over and that you are safe. Review the pain event a second time. After you have completed the second review, go through the experience one more time, this time in reverse. Start at the moment in the present time when you know that the experience is over and that you are safe, then go backwards in time through the experiences you have recalled until you reach the moment just before your pain began or got worse. When you feel ready, open your eyes, stretch your body, and gather together what you have learned. Write down your discoveries in your own journal or notebook, or on a special bookmark for this chapter.

Healing Your Heart Pain

The energy field around your heart is one of the most powerful in the body. Researchers have noted that the heart seems to be the entry point for the energy in the rest of the body; it provides the biggest natural pendulum in the energy system; and it has the strongest oscillation.

Taking the information you have just received about your heart pain from the exercises above, prepare to experience a healing meditation for your heart using your breath and sensory imagery. As before, read through the exercise first. If helpful, record the script so that you can concentrate on listening. Make sure you have your journal or notebook ready at the end to record your experience.

Exercise: **Breathing through Your Heart**[6]

Imagine that you can breathe through your heart. Imagine that you can breathe right into the center of your heart . . . aware of its rhythm . . . your whole body can begin to breathe with the steady rhythm of your heart. Maybe you can even feel the air around you begin to pulse, your whole body pulsing this rhythm, creating a force field of energy all around you. . . . You might want to let your arms rest somewhere on your body so that you can feel the rise and fall of your breath. As you continue to feel the flow of air move in and out, you might even feel a tingling in the air around you and the gentle vibration of energy on your skin, as if you were surrounded and protected by a soft pillow of energy insulating you from whatever you don't need or want, yet allowing you to take in whatever is nourishing to you. Can you feel a growing radiance move through your heart?

Now imagine that you can feel all the moments of love and kindness that have ever been felt for you, even those you have not been aware of. . . . Feel your energy field pulling in all the lovingkindness, every prayer and good wish and message of love that has ever been sent your way, all of it filling the energy field around your heart and all the rest of you . . . feel it coming in as if to a powerful magnet. Maybe you can sense this love as a calming presence, a soft weight, a gentle hand on your shoulder, a loving voice, an animal, a guardian angel, sweet spirits and guides.

Some of these messengers of love may be known to you, some perhaps completely unknown. It doesn't matter what you find . . . you can feel their protection and support, breathing it into your heart, breathing it into your body, letting it fill you, all that caring, all that love, feeling the love spreading through the body, gently pulsing out from the center of your heart, moving through you, like ripples through a pond. . . .

Gently with soft eyes, come back into the room, knowing in a deep place that you have received something important, something profoundly healing. . . . Take a few moments now to sense the completion of this healing for now . . . then when you are ready, begin to move and stretch, letting your eyes open with a soft focus and noticing how the world around you seems different now, and how your inner world might also seem different.

Take a few moments to reorient to the room around you. If you'd like, record your observations and feelings in your notebook or journal.

Healing Suffering

Suffering is defined as the experience of physical or psychological pain and distress. Many factors can contribute to suffering. First, we can develop negative beliefs about ourselves during the course of a pain condition that increase our degree of suffering. For example, we can decide that we are being punished because our pain persists with such unrelenting intensity. We can decide that we are helpless to recover from our pain, or that perhaps we don't deserve to resolve our pain condition. These negative beliefs may build on those we developed in childhood, often as a result of early traumatic experiences, and therefore they are so deeply engrained that we feel "that's just the way it is."

Is there really no gain without pain? It may be true that physical pain can sometimes help us become aware of the more global pain that results from imbalance in our greater lives. This does *not* mean, however, that a chronic pain condition has developed in order to "teach us a lesson."

When we suffer, we want to find someone to blame, even if it is ourselves. The contemporary focus on personal responsibility for our life circumstances frequently can be funneled into what has been called "New Age guilt." Not only is this not helpful, it is not accurate because chronic pain consists of so many different dimensions that include genetics, injury caused by others, invasive medical procedures for treatment, and unique life circumstances.

A balanced view is best. Once chronic pain has developed, we can decide to learn from the pain as part of our healing. If we are given lemons, we might as well make lemonade! So frequently although we do not have a choice about the pain condition that plagues us, we do have a choice about how we decide to relate to the pain.

As Steven Levine points out, healing our suffering means not so much the absence of pain but the ability to meet it with love and compassion instead of blame, fear, and loathing. It is the ability to enter those areas of ourselves from which we have withdrawn with fear and helplessness, bringing mercy and lovingkindness.

Sometimes our suffering comes from a loss of meaning in our lives or a loss of connection with God, however you conceive of the divine power. Where is God when we hurt? Our pain pilgrimage may help us realize that it is not God who is absent or dead but that we are.

One of my patients, suffering from fibromyalgia, chronic fatigue, and migraine headaches, was struggling to heal some of the emotional abandonment and terror from her childhood. When we talked about the possibility of using God or her higher power as a resource, she commented, "When I'm in that black place, I don't have the strength or the faith to reach out to God. I'm not sure God exists during those times." It was important for her to discover that God could find her—all she had to do was ask. If we believe that God is love, then there is no limit to the healing that can take place.

Steven Levine has written that there are three stages to the healing of sorrow: 1) We must soften to our pain. That is, we must open ourselves to the willingness of knowing our grief rather than banishing it from our awareness. 2) We must cultivate kindness and forgiveness toward ourselves and have the courage to send love to ourselves *especially because we are in pain*. 3) The last stage is acceptance or making peace with our sorrow or suffering.

It is especially important since we carry suffering in our bodies to forgive our bodies for our suffering. We often feel betrayed by our bodies and so have banished or exiled various parts of them. It is especially powerful, then, to soften our hearts into forgiveness for our bodies.

Exercise: Loving Your Body through Pain

Pause for a moment. Imagine the part of the body that seems to create the most pain for you—your foot, your pelvis, your hip joint, your neck. Think about this part of your body as a vulnerable, weak, struggling part of you, raw with pain. Send messages of acceptance and love to this wounded part of you. How does this part respond? What messages does it send in return?

What About Forgiveness?

Many toxic emotions are the result of wounds we have received from others. Yet most of us resist forgiveness because doing so might remove our feelings of hurt and betrayal. Refusing to forgive cuts us off from interpersonal love and growth and any hope of resolving the conflict or hurt.

Janis Abram Spring has written that genuine forgiveness is possible only when both parties involved in a wounding experience are willing to contribute equally to the healing process. When this is not possible, the alternative is **acceptance.** Spring defines acceptance as a program of caring for the self through generous gifts of love and healing. This is accomplished by the self and for the self and asks nothing of the other person.

Spring identifies ten steps in acceptance[7] that might be helpful to consider:

1. Honor the full range of your feelings—rage, hurt, despair, etc.
2. Give up the need for revenge but seek a fair resolution

3. Stop obsessing about the injury and reengage with life
4. Protect yourself from further abuse or injury
5. View the offender's behavior in terms of his/her own limitations
6. Look honestly at your own contributions to the problem
7. Challenge your false assumptions about what happened
8. Look at the offender objectively, weighing strengths against weaknesses
9. Decide carefully what relationship is possible with the offender that would be healthy for you
10. Forgive yourself for your own shortcomings

Exercise: **Walk through the Door of Forgiveness**[8]

Now that you have considered some ways of healing suffering and Janis Spring's steps of forgiveness, you may be ready to engage in a forgiveness practice to create some closure to a painful relationship.

Imagine or think about a beautiful hallway with several closed doors. In a few moments, your intuition will lead you toward one of these doors. When you are ready, allow yourself to be drawn inside. Behind the door will be a person connected to a painful experience in your past. Notice your surroundings once you cross over the threshold. Spend time expressing all of your feelings about what happened between you; acknowledge your appreciations for the person's strengths as well as awareness of their limitations; look at your own contributions to the problem and forgive yourself for your shortcomings.

Tell the person what kind of relationship you feel is possible given all that has happened between you. Discuss the way you will relate in the future. Take all the time that is needed and then say goodbye to the old relationship. When you are ready, step back through the doorway and into the hallway. Leave the past relationship behind you. How do you feel as you step into the hallway and begin walking in a different direction?

What has shifted? Try this exercise any time feelings of resentment or obsessive thoughts resurface. How do your feelings of suffering change over time? You may want to write about this experience in your pain notebook or diary.

SUMMARY: This chapter considered the role of emotional pain or distress in chronic pain conditions. You reflected on five ways that physical and emotional pain are the same in terms of our biological responses, and you explored several ways of healing your heart pain and suffering, including breathing through the heart and practicing loving self-forgiveness. This chapter concludes with the midline meridian protocol from Energy Psychology to practice clearing a combination of physical and emotional distress.

Body Awareness Skill #9

LOVE: Clearing Emotional and Physical Pain

For this skill, we go back to the realm of Energy Psychology that we first visited in Chapter Six. This protocol, originally developed by Fred Gallo,[9] is called the midline technique. I have found it especially effective in neutralizing intense states of emotional and physical feelings. There are only four treatment points involved, and each can be tapped, rubbed, or touched. Again, as with other energy protocols, this approach is very gentle and will not worsen your feelings. You may notice only subtle change at first, but with practice your results will increase. You may want to review the energy boosters from Chapter Six before you start.

1. First, use the three boosters to create a positive energy field:
   a. Drink lots of water.
   b. Correct for energy disorganization with the overenergy correction:
      • While sitting, place left ankle over right;

- *Extend arms in front of the body with backs of hands touching;*
- *Bring right hand over left and clasp fingers together;*
- *Fold arms and rest hands under chin;*
- *Rest tongue against palate of mouth behind top of front teeth;*
- *Breathe for 1–2 minutes with eyes and mouth closed.*

c. *Create a positive energy field. Rub or hold the sore spots which are one inch below your left and right collarbone notches and three to four inches toward your shoulder while affirming out loud three or more times: "I deeply and completely love and appreciate myself even though I have this reaction (or feeling or symptom)." Make sure that you resonate fully with the wording you choose.*

Let's say you choose to clear anger toward someone who has betrayed you. Your affirmation might be: "I deeply and completely love and accept myself even though I have this anger toward _____." Then add other negative beliefs you want to be free of: "I deeply and completely love and accept myself even though . . . I believe I can't change this anger . . . I believe it's impossible to be over this anger . . . I feel guilt and shame about having this anger . . . I believe I can't do what's necessary to resolve this anger," etc.

2. *While thinking about the combination of distressing physical and emotional feelings related to your anger, stimulate the four primary treatment points of the midline protocol (see the diagram on page 119): TE (third eye point between the eyebrows), UN (under the nose), UL (under the lip), and CH (on the middle of the chest). Hold or rub or tap each point for as long as feels helpful. Notice what is happening in your body and keep stimulating a particular point as long as there is a helpful response. Make sure to breathe at least one full cycle before moving to the next point.*

3. *If progress remains incomplete, you may add other points further down the midline (e.g. 3 inches above the navel, 2 inches above the navel, 1 inch above the navel), or you may return to the most powerful of the*

*four points for you, or repeat all four points again. Some people improve results by holding one hand across the occipital ridge at the back of the head while stimulating the midline points. If you feel stuck, you may also want to correct for possible reversals using an affirmation such as "I deeply love and accept myself even though I **still** have **some** of this anger," etc. Say this out loud while stimulating the sore spot on your left chest, or while tapping on the side of the hand "karate chop" point. Then go through the steps above a second time.*

4. *Tune back in to your original emotional/physical pain response. What number would you give it now out of a 10-point scale? Has it changed since the beginning of this protocol? If so, how would you describe the change?*

If you use this protocol once or twice a day for several days you will notice a significant change in the targeted problem you started with. Make some written or mental notes about the changes you find.

Before you go on to the final chapter, spend a little time reflecting on your experience of this chapter on heart pain. Do you feel more loving and accepting of yourself? Do you feel softer toward others who may have hurt you in the past?

CHAPTER TEN

Build on Success
When You Haven't Got Time for the Pain

During this last chapter, we will review all the tools you have worked with in this book, giving you an opportunity to pull together the material you have been introduced to with an eye to future learning. I hope you will continue to use the material presented here as a resource to help you on your continued pilgrimage of recovery and transformation.

And, if you haven't yet jelled what you learned into a step-by-step personal pain protocol, you will have a chance now to put together your own rapid, reliable formula for pain relief.

Review

This opening section presents a streamlined version of what you have encountered during your reading experience. Each point below links all the concepts and techniques in each particular chapter so that you can easily retrieve them for a more expanded overview. Of course, as always, you are also invited to work out your very own format for review.

At the beginning of this book, we affirmed the importance of bringing your mind awareness together with body experience to create a powerful mind-body partnership that can reverse the course of your pain condition. The ten body awareness building blocks provide the framework for our review.

1. The first body awareness skill for reversing the course of chronic pain is to *be with your body and breathe*. The pain gate system teaches us that:

   - Competing sensations such as gentle pressure, soothing massage, topical analgesics, and different types of breathing can actually block the transmission of many pain sensations, closing the gates in the dorsal horn so that pain sensations are not relayed on to the brain.

   - Imagery and other ways of stimulating the brain, such as exercise, can generate positive chemistry to counteract the pain sensations that may have already been allowed to move through the gates to your brain.

   - There is no single medication, person, or technique that will remove your pain. Throughout this book, we have emphasized that chronic pain is a complex, multi-dimensional condition, and therefore requires multiple interventions including body-focused therapy, medication, developing a positive mental and spiritual focus, use of supplements and nutrition, and the ability to regulate your daily rhythms.

   - And, most of all, reversing the course of chronic or persistent pain involves learning to use your body's wisdom and your felt-body sense.

   - You practiced different types of breathing including the *calming breath* (breathing in and out through your nose), *foursquare breathing* (inhale for a count of four, hold for four, exhale four, and hold for four), *circular breathing*, and the *purifying breath* (send healing light through your body as you inhale, and release what is no longer needed as you exhale).

2. The second body awareness skill is to *feel your body* in order to begin regulating your pain levels. Several strategies were presented:

- Observing your pain from a distance;
- Focusing on the *felt sense* of body sensations, including pleasure, that surround your pain;
- Adjusting your daily rhythms so that you find the best arrangement for exercise, self-treatment, relaxation, and enjoyment;
- Self-massage In a bath or pulsing shower;
- Pendulation.

3. The third body awareness skill taught you to intervene early in your pain cycle to achieve *reliable relaxation* rather than waiting until you are in severe pain and then trying to relax. Resources for relaxation include the following:
   - Herb Benson's relaxation response, a structured way of relaxing each group of muscles starting with your feet and moving up to your head.
   - Several suggestions to achieve reliable relaxation: a) Intervene early in small steps; b) keep it simple; c) find pleasure and enjoyment; d) create a relaxation practice that truly relaxes mind, heart, spirit, as well as body—a practice that all of you says "yes" to; e) trust your body's wisdom by paying attention to natural feedback to discover what your body likes and what it says "no" to; f) use pendulation to begin to create new responses in your body.
   - The tension release method of progressive relaxation—tightening the muscles in different areas of your body starting with one foot, holding the tension as you hold your breath, then releasing the muscles along with your breath. Options provide for focus on a few body areas easy for you to tense-relax, small areas or large ones, and putting all your stress or discomfort in a tightened fist or marble and then gradually letting go.

4. The fourth body awareness skill is *imagine*—learning to tap the creative imagination to bring relief to your body and a different pain reality. You learned three types of imagery:

- *Conflict-free imagery* captures an experience that is free of anxiety, stress, pain, or any internal conflict or hurt.
- *The Circle of Pain image* gathers all of your pain into a brightly colored circle. You play with the circle in your mind's eye, making it gigantic, then shrinking it down to a tiny dot. Imagine that the circle eventually becomes a balloon and floats up and away from you until it is no longer in sight.
- *The Brain's Pain Relief Center* invites you to take a special journey through your body as a miniature version of yourself. The miniature self moves with the breath to explore pain areas with a powerful microscope or camera, then moves to the brain's pain regulation center to create whatever is needed—an internal IV drip, a special foam to cool or relax, or a special internal sleeve or sock to cushion, etc.

5. The fifth body awareness skill involves *mindfulness and spirituality*. One aspect of spirituality is exploration of the power of positive intention ("I want to be more loving toward myself"), as well as the power of attention to the fullness of the mind in the current moment through prayer and meditation practice. Strategies include:
   - The body scan to be with your felt sense in the moment.
   - Sensory Awareness Training through the "4-3-2-1" exercise, starting with the awareness of four external images, four external sounds, four external feelings, then three, two, and one. Then with eyes closed, find four *internal* images, four internal sensations, and four internal sounds, then three, two, and one.
   - Inner strength to connect you with the divine energy of your essence, the energy inside that has helped you survive and prevail over many difficult circumstances
   - Lovingkindness or *metta* meditation that starts with loving messages for self then evolves into sending loving messages to others.

- The use of personal prayer.
- Mindfulness meditation practice that features the concept of beginner's mind, gathering all your awareness as you breathe in, holding your awareness as you hold your breath, then letting all of this go as you exhale. With the next breath in, you move into a new moment (as if for the very first time) and then repeat the practice.

6. The sixth body awareness skill encourages you to *energize* as an important part of healing pain. You practiced:
- The Three Boosters: 1) Drink water to get your energy moving; 2) Do the overenergy correction to rebalance the energy system (see page 109); and 3) Create a positive energy field by correcting energy reversals that are the opposite of your positive intentions to resolve your pain using the affirmation approach.
- The TAT helps to gently release the tyranny of pain triggers.
- The eight-point protocol (EFT) helps clear different aspects of pain. After completing the Three Boosters (see above), you choose a reminder phrase such as "My fear of more pain." Repeat the reminder phrase as you touch each point, then take at least a full breath in and out before moving to the next point (see page 119 for the eight points). If your pain number is not close to zero when you finish, repeat the protocol with a more relevant reminder phrase, or complete the energy sandwich by adding a brain balancer and then stimulate the eight points again.
- Daily energy practice: The Three Thumps to help you with mental clarity and alertness, the overenergy correction as a stress reducer, and positive affirmations related to specific energy reversals.

7. Body awareness skill #7 directs you to *make the right moves* for your body. Ideally, by now you employ some type of regular exercise and physical movement every day, including warm-ups,

stretching, and heating and icing as needed. And perhaps you have become more appreciative of the value of physical touch to bring comfort, such as that found in regular massage or other bodywork. In this chapter you also practiced the following:

- Self-Massage: Bringing pleasure to those parts of your body that are sensitive and sore with soft, slow, gentle touch. The lightest touch without any movement at all can bring a sense of connection with the parts that are hurting. You may have enjoyed the shower massage (see page 31) as an alternative, or have learned to work with your trigger points.

- Seeking Your Inner Coach: You created an inner coach, mentor, or trainer by thinking of an actual coach who has been helpful to you, a friend who has an attitude you would like to emulate, or a former therapist or mentor with whom you have worked. At this point, can you ask your coach for help with motivation, for encouragement, or guidance with pain-free movement when you need it?

8. The eighth body awareness skill is to *heal the trauma–pain connection through pendulation*. Our nervous system has three possibilities when we are confronted with a perceived threat to our survival: freeze, fight, and flight. You now know that these trauma responses can create a roller coaster of pain when you are reminded of a threat, past or present. To reverse the chronic pain cycle, it is essential that you learn to find and "thaw" the patterns of frozen constriction in your body. To do this we explored:

- Pendulation: First, you use a body scan to explore sensations connected to constriction including tightness, tension, and pain. After gently exploring the edges of these constricted areas and then finding relatively more expanded areas in your body, your breath becomes the bridge between expansion and constriction to dissolve the link between discomfort and past trauma.

- Inner cooperation involves envisioning the part of you that seems to create conflict related to pain or that resists healing. The next step is finding help for this part, perhaps through the Inner Table technique, where all your parts (including your inner coach) can join together to help resolve conflicts that are barriers to recovery.

9. The ninth body awareness skill is *love*—learning to embrace the heart of your pain problem, which involves healing emotional pain. You explored what Steven Levine calls "unattended sorrow" or feelings of grief, anger, and betrayal related to loss. Ideally, you have considered specific types of unresolved emotional pain that might be related to your physical pain. Forgiveness and acceptance are particularly important. Perhaps you have learned to do some of the following:

   • Love your body through pain: Can you send loving and healing messages to the parts of your body that seem to create the most pain for you? What difference has this made so far?

   • Walk through the Door of Forgiveness: Use this exercise to heal the pain of a relationship that disappointed or hurt you.

   • Clear emotional and physical pain states using the energy midline meridian technique. While focusing on some combination of physical or emotional pain, you stimulated each of four treatment points (see page 119). Remember to breathe while rubbing, tapping, or holding each point and notice any subtle changes that take place.

10. The final of the ten building blocks, presented in this chapter, reminds you to *build on success* to create your own pain protocol or step-by-step prescription for pain relief and regulation. Throughout this book, you have been urged to listen to your body's biofeedback, to choose the tools that most fully resonate with you, and then to practice creating results that are sustained across time before adding any additional strategies.

As you continue to explore the world of pain self-treatment after finishing this book, you will keep adding steps to your protocol to create a chain of positive changes that translate into successful self-management and reversal of the effects of persistent or chronic pain.

Build Your Own Pain Protocol

Now that you have reached the end of this book, it is crucial to combine the best of the approaches you have explored into a step-by-step formula so that you have a recipe for reliable relief of emotional and physical pain. When your pain levels are high, it is hard to focus or think about what you have learned. What seems to work well is to choose a few methods at one time to work with, and make sure you practice them in the order that brings you optimal results.

Start with the key words BREATHE, FEEL, and RELIABLE RELAXATION from the first three chapters. The skill exercises may have already helped you to develop a sequence that you are practicing.

↶ JOE

Joe has pain in his lower back from a herniated disc. The three-step self-treatment method he selected from the exercises for the first three chapters was:
1. Cleansing breath + body sanctuary
2. Pendulate between pain sensations and areas of expansion in the body
3. The marble method

Joe practiced these three steps of his protocol twice a day, once when he first arrived at work and again at the end of the day when he returned home. He found that practicing the cleansing breath method and becoming aware of his inner sanctuary helped him to settle into his body, then he could pendulate between the more positive sensations and the sensations of pain. Finally, he employed the marble method to send any remaining back pain into a small stone and feel the discomfort releasing as he squeezed the stone and then let go.

Stop and ask yourself, what can *you* put together from the first three chapters?

Next, think about IMAGERY, MINDFULNESS, and ENERGIZ- ING. You might want to start by thinking about what aspects of these skills you are already using in your everyday life. Again, Joe's story may help you.

The first three steps helped Joe lower his pain levels from an aver- age of 8 to between 6 and 7. To get more results, he practiced with the "Brain's Pain Relief System" imagery and sent the miniature ver- sion of himself into the area of pain and inflammation dressed as a firefighter who used cooling foam to bring down the swelling and soreness. He then sent the "firefighter" into the brain's control room to turn on an internal IV of "toredol," the pain medication that had most helped him after surgery. He set a timer so that this imagined medication would drip into the painful area of his back for the time period that he needed an extra boost.

In working further with the skills found in this book, Joe learned that spirituality was an important part of his healing. This surprised him because he never went to church and was uncomfortable with the idea of "God." Yet he found a spiritual home in the practice of mindfulness. He learned to practice witnessing all of his thoughts, feelings, and body sensations, using his breath to hold them and then letting go as he exhaled. He found that a 10-minute practice during his lunch hour allowed him to stay centered and be more productive.

From the energy tradition, Joe found the overenergy correction to be the most effective practice for him. Because he was slow to get going in the morning, he found that 2–3 minutes of practicing this method while he waited for his coffee to perk, followed by the Three Thumps, was the best combination to get his energy moving for the day.

So, using the first six building blocks, Joe's protocol looked like this:

1. Overenergy exercise + the Three Thumps in the morning before coffee.
2. Cleansing breath & body sanctuary + pendulation + the marble relaxation method for 5–10 minutes or so when he first arrived at work and as a transition between work and settling in at home for the evening.
3. During most lunch hours, Joe closed his door and practiced at least 10 minutes of mindfulness. Whenever his pain level spiked during the day, he practiced using the brain's pain relief system imagery to move his pain numbers back down the scale.

What about MOVING, PENDULATION, and bringing LOVE to emotional pain? You may already have a good working protocol drawn from the first six building blocks. Yet it's important not to forget exercise, one of the best sources of pleasurable feelings and the best way of cultivating strength and resiliency in your body. Nor should you forget the regular practice of pendulum methods to help reset your nervous system to turn off alarm and fear reactions. And, if you have unresolved emotional pain that continues to trigger or increase pain levels, you must find a way to heal any emotional suffering. How can you add these elements to your self-treatment practice?

Joe was doing quite well with the self-treatment formula described above. This gave shape to his day and helped him measure regular practice in reversing his pain condition. As he felt more in control of his back pain, he began to exercise more regularly. At first he returned to the stretches that had been recommended by his physical therapist during regular breaks in his workday. Next, Joe added water walking and aerobics at the gym and bicycling on the stationary bike. Whenever he had any soreness after exercise periods, he faithfully practiced pendulation between feelings of strength and vitality that resulted from moving his body, and his awareness of any discomfort or stiffness.

Emotional pain was harder for him to deal with. In fact, Joe was very resistant to any suggestions I made to him. One day, however, he came to my office and told me that at a family gathering over the weekend, he noticed that following a brief disagreement with his father while they were barbecuing steaks, his back pain began to increase. This was the first time he made the emotional pain–body pain connection. He found the Door of Forgiveness exercise very helpful in letting go of old hurts with his father and realized that he could actually enjoy family gatherings rather than dreading or avoiding them.

So Joe's protocol ended up like this:

1. Overenergy exercise + the Three Thumps in the morning before coffee.
2. Cleansing breath & body sanctuary + pendulation + the marble relaxation method for 5–10 minutes or so when he first arrived at work and as a transition between work and settling in at home for the evening.
3. Mindfulness during lunch hours and use of the "brain's control room" imagery whenever his pain spiked during the day.
4. Strengthening his back and the rest of his body during workouts at the gym three days a week, and pendulation whenever he experienced residual soreness.
5. The Door of Forgiveness and other ways of healing emotional

pain were used as needed, usually after a time when Joe noticed the emotional-physical pain connection.

Still stumped as to what your self-treatment protocol might be? Maybe Nancy's protocol below will give you further hints.

↩ NANCY

Nancy developed carpal tunnel syndrome and tendonitis in both arms due to the word processing required by her job as a paralegal with a large real estate law firm. She had difficulty being in her body and was uncomfortable with the breathing techniques and various attempts to discover her felt sense. She also found imagery unhelpful because she felt pressured to "come up with something" and so resisted practicing. However, she did find beneficial the idea of using a pain notebook to track her daily pain levels to prevent spikes from happening, which always discouraged her and set her back. She learned to use her body's "yes and no" responses to help her regulate her activity levels and keep pain from spiraling out of control.

She was able to develop reliable relaxation through yoga classes and pickup soccer games at the neighborhood playing field. We added icing of her arms following all exercise and at work during times of high stress before deadlines.

Although the energy techniques seemed effective for her, Nancy felt silly doing them so she didn't. But mindfulness was very useful in clearing her mind of negative thoughts and fear reactions. She bought a Jon Kabat-Zinn CD and listened to it during her mid-day break at the office.

Nancy's pain protocol looked like this:
1. Pain notebook and tracking daily pain levels;
2. Reliable daily relaxation through yoga classes and soccer followed by stretches and icing;

3. Almost daily practice of mindfulness meditation using a CD recording to guide her;
4. Icing her arms when her pain increased, after returning home from work, and just before bed.

If you compare Joe's protocol with Nancy's, you might conclude that Joe probably accomplished more because he used more tools than Nancy. But I guess that depends on how you measure success.

Nancy was told that she might have to have surgery on one or both arms. After six months of working with the tools she selected, her pain levels had dropped to 4 or 5 from an average of 8 when she started working with the program in this book. Her doctor told her if she maintained or even increased her progress, she would not need surgery. Nancy also began to "forget" to take her pain medications where previously she had felt desperate for each dose. Maybe comparisons aren't relevant. Both Joe and Nancy have found permanent relief using very different paths.

Trust Your Body to Teach You How to Get Out of Pain

Ideally you have learned the importance of trusting your body's wisdom as you worked your way through this book. Your body is the best teacher and healer you will ever encounter. All of the techniques and tools presented in *Reversing Chronic Pain* are designed to help you tip the scales of your daily experience away from unending, unchanging pain and toward health, wholeness, and well-being. Developing a trusting partnership between mind and body is a lifelong task. I hope you feel closer to that goal than you did when you first picked up this book.

Body Awareness Skill #10

BUILD ON SUCCESS: Keep Learning from Your Body

Please continue to use these materials for future learning. You may find that parts of this book do not resonate as much as others on your first reading. Coming back to the body awareness skills after using your initial pain prescription for an interval of time may lead you into skill areas that weren't of interest or did not seem possible for you to approach before.

Each time you work your way through this book, you will become more mindful of your own resilience and the vast resources contained in joining your mind awareness with your body experience, bringing mindful attention to your spiritual needs, and releasing past emotional hurts.

And, of course, there are many more techniques and models[1] to explore beyond this book. Each of them offers unique opportunities for you to partner body and mind to end the reign of pain in your life. You have my very best wishes as you continue to embark on this exciting and challenging pilgrimage to a place of wholeness and health.

Appendix 1
THE TOP 20 SUPPLEMENTS FOR PAIN RELIEF

In his book *The Chronic Pain Solution*, on pp. 138–147, author James Dillard lists his top 20 supplements for pain relief, the neurotransmitters they impact, and the specific pain conditions they help. These are:

Multivitamins (overall toning)

B-complex vitamins (peripheral neuropathy)

Bromelain (chronic sprains and strains)

Calcium (headaches, nerve pain, pelvic pain including PMS)

Capsaicin or capsicum (*topical only*; for peripheral, joint, and nerve pain) [May reduce substance P, a neurotransmitter that facilitates the spread of pain messages]

Devil's claw (osteoarthritis, other types of arthritis, tendonitis)

Feverfew (may prevent migraines)

Fish oil (any pain; inflammatory disorders)

Gamma-Linolenic Acid (GLA) (inflammatory arthritis, pelvic pain, any inflammation)

Ginger (inflammatory arthritis, nausea and other effects of pain medication)

Glucosamine and chondroitin (osteoarthritis)

Kava (anxiety, insomnia, muscle tension)

Magnesium (headaches, chronic muscle spasm, leg cramps, peripheral neuropathy, any nerve pain)

Quercetin (arthritis)

St. John's wort (depression) [may help boost serotonin; higher levels of serotonin are associated with reduced depression, insomnia, and pain]

Turmeric (inflammatory arthritis, other inflammatory conditions)

Valerian (insomnia, muscle pain)

Vitamin B_2 (Migraines)

White Willow (low back pain)

Because some of these supplements are considered controversial by the Federal Drug Administration, it is important to discuss your use of them and monitor their effects with your treating physician.

Appendix 2
RESOURCES

Academy for Guided Imagery (AGI)
30765 Pacific Coast Highway
Suite 369
Malibu, CA 90265
TEL: 800.726.2070
FAX: 800.727.2070
www.academyforguidedimagery.com

American Academy of Medical Acupuncture
4929 Wilshire Boulevard
Suite 428
Los Angeles, CA 90010
TEL: 323.937.5514
http://www.medicalacupuncture.org/acu_info/index.html
See the website page: "Find an acupuncturist near you"

American Academy of Pain Management
13947 Mono Way #A
Sonora, CA 95370
TEL: 209.533.9744
FAX: 209.533.9750
aapm@aapainmanage.org
http://www.aapainmanage.org/links/Links.php
http://www.aapainmanage.org/search/FacilSearch.php

American Chronic Pain Association
PO Box 850
Rocklin, CA 95677
TEL: 800.533.3231
FAX: 916.632.3208
ACPA@pacbell.net
See the website pages: "Preparing for your Doctor"
"A Consumer Guide to Options for Managing Chronic Pain"

American Pain Foundation
201 North Charles Street, Suite 710
Baltimore, MD 21201-4111
TEL: 888.615.7246
info@painfoundation.org
http://www.painfoundation.org/
See especially the website pages: "Pain Information Library"
"Q&A about Pain"
"Useful Links about Pain"
"Pain Resource Indicator"
"Online Advocacy Center"

American Pain Society
4700 West Lake Avenue
Glenview, IL 60025
TEL: 847.375.8758
FAX: 877.734.8759
info@ampainsoc.org
http://www.ampainsoc.org/people/
See links to resources with people in pain

American Society of Clinical Hypnosis
140 N. Bloomingdale Road
Bloomingdale, IL 60108

TEL: 640.980.4740
info@asch.net
http://asch.net/
http://asch.net/referrals.as
http://asch.net/genpubinfo.htm

Association for Comprehensive Energy Psychology (ACEP)
PO Box 910244
San Diego, CA 92191-0244
TEL: 619.861.2237
FAX: 760.804.3704
http://www.energypsych.org

Eye Movement Desensitization and Reprocessing International Association (EMDRIA)
5806 Mesa Drive
Suite 360
Austin, Texas 78731
TEL: 512.451.5200
FAX: 512.451.5256
info@emdria.org
www.emdria.org

Foundation for Human Enrichment (Somatic Experiencing)
7102 La Vista Place
Suite 200
Niwot, CO 80503
TEL: 303.652.4035
FAX: 303.652.4039
info@traumahealing.com
www.traumahealing.com/registry.html
http://www.traumahealing.com/registry.html

Milton H. Erickson Foundation
3606 North 24th Street
Phoenix, AZ 85016
TEL: 602.956.6196
FAX: 602.956.0519
http://www.erickson-foundation.org/

National Institute for the Clinical Applications of Behavioral
Medicine (NICABM)
PO Box 523
Mansfield Center, CT 06250
TEL: 800.743.2226
FAX: 800.423.4512
information@nicabm.com
www.nicabm.com

WEB PAGES

Academy of Guided Imagery: www.interactiveimagery.com
Donna Eden and David Feinstein: www.Innersource.com
Emotional Freedom Technique (EFT): www.emofree.com
Eye Movement Desensitization and Reprocessing Association
   (EMDR): www.emdria.org
Tapas Fleming: www.tat-intl.com
Fred Gallo, PhD: http://www.energypsych.com/
Peter Levine: www.traumahealing.com
Belleruth Naparstek: http://www.healthjourneys.com/
Pat Ogden: www.sensorimotorpsychotherapy.org
Maggie Phillips, Ph.D.: http://www.maggiephillipsphd.com
Thought Field Therapy (TFT): www.tftrx.com

Notes

INTRODUCTION

1. The term "tipping point" refers to a popular book, *The Tipping Point*, by Malcolm Gladwell (New York: Little, Brown, & Co., 2002). The author makes the point that a single ill person can start an epidemic of a disease, and that as it gains momentum, it can begin either to "stick" by having a dramatic impact, or continue to keep changing, evolving into other forms, therefore diffusing its negative impact. In *Reversing Chronic Pain*, we will consider both what "tips" toward greater relief and freedom from pain, as well as how to make strategies "stick" for a lasting impact against pain.

2. "Persistent pain" is a relatively new term for pain that persists even though the source of the pain has resolved, or has healed to the point that the physical cause of the pain is no longer an issue. You'll be learning more about this in Chapter One. If persistent pain cannot be reversed, a chronic pain condition can result.

CHAPTER ONE

1. Two books that make this point are *The Psychobiology of Mindbody Healing* by Ernest Rossi (New York: W.W. Norton, 1997), and Candace Pert's *Molecules of Emotion* (New York: Scribner, 2002).

2. Melzack and Wall describe their gate theory in their new book, *Textbook of Pain* (2005), but perhaps a more readable discussion can be found in their earlier book, *The Challenge of Pain* (New York: Bantam, 2004).

3. An excellent discussion of nerve pain can be found at http://www.spine-health.com/topics/cd/neuropain/neuropain03.html as well as through many other websites.

4. There is some research indicating that dull pain or itching travels

0.5–2.0 miles per second; sharp or burning pain travels 5–35 miles per second, and soothing touch travels 35–75 miles per second. James Dillard presents this material in *The Chronic Pain Solution* (New York: Bantam, 2002), p. 33.

5. A good guide to the use of capsaicin can be found in James Dillard's *The Chronic Pain Solution*, pp. 139–140.

6. A complete guide to the treatment of inflammation is *The Inflammation Syndrome* by Jack Challem (New York: Wiley, 2003).

7. These four neurotransmitters appear to be the most important in their effects within the pain system. To learn more about them, consult Dillard's *The Chronic Pain Solution*, pp. 37–39 (see note 4).

8. For example, omega-3 oils found in deep-water fish, walnuts, and flaxseed can inhibit the production of neurotransmitters such as substance P and bradykinins, which are believed to increase pain and inflammation. Adding green leafy vegetables, such as broccoli, spinach, and chard, provides a strong source of B-complex vitamins, often diminished in pain conditions caused by damaged or misfiring nerves. Green leafy vegetables also contain high amounts of magnesium, which helps relax smooth muscles and may reduce stress and inflammation.

   It is important to note that specific foods may be toxic for you. Allergies to food and other environmental toxins can create inflammation. You may want to explore your body's reactions to wheat, dairy, corn, soy, eggs, citrus, and other common irritants. Consulting a nutritionist who specializes in food issues with chronic health problems may be helpful in determining foods that could be added to or deleted from your diet. Again, consult James Dillard's book, *The Chronic Pain Solution*, pp. 125–136 (see note 4).

9. The AIDS cocktail gives us a model for how to heal challenging, overwhelming health problems such as chronic pain. When no one intervention does the job, the best approach is to combine the most powerful or "active" ingredients. This combination approach works because the effect is greater than the sum of various individual ingredients. You will learn how to use this approach throughout the book.

10. Melzack and Wall include an excellent section on the control of pain (see pp. 195–261, and note 2 above).

11. Nutrients that increase serotonin are usually found in foods that contain L-tryptophan, including green leafy vegetables, turkey, whole grains, or fresh, low-fat dairy foods. See Dillard for a brief discussion on pp. 125–149 (see note 4 above). If your diet already follows these guidelines, you may need to boost serotonin levels through use of an SSRI antidepressant such as Zoloft.

12. Another approach is the S-M-A-R-T model for setting goals. S = focus on specific behaviors; M = measurable change; A = attainable progress (you know you can do it); R = realistic (it makes sense for where you are); and T = the goal is **tangible** and **timely.** You can get more information through http://www.goal-setting-guide.com/smart-goals.html.

13. This scale (0 = no pain; 10 = maximum pain) is one of the best measures of your pain levels. We really have no technology as yet that can measure pain levels with any accuracy. So our best measure is your own pain "sense."

14. Research in the area of biofeedback has concluded that relaxation training alone is as effective as biofeedback for tension and migraine headaches, lower back pain, and other common pain conditions. See Melzack and Wall (note 2), p. 247.

15. The term "relaxation response" was first used by Herb Benson, a medical researcher at Harvard. In his book, *The Relaxation Response* (New York: Consumer Reports Books, 1993), he details the natural relaxation response created by the nervous system and how to turn it on through such practices as yoga, meditation, and self-hypnosis.

16. The first three breathing techniques are found in Dillard, pp. 110–112 (see note 4).

CHAPTER TWO

1. *Turning Suffering Inside Out* (Boston: Shambhala, 2000) by Darlene Cohen is an excellent book about the emotional suffering related to pain. The quotation can be found on page 39.

2. These emotional and physical pain categories are presented in Margaret Caudill's book, *Managing Pain Before it Manages You* (New York: Guilford, 2002), p. 11.

3. Eugene Gendlin wrote the classic book, *Focusing* (New York: Bantam,

1982), based on his research at the University of Chicago. Gendlin and his colleagues and students studied hundreds of hours of psychotherapy sessions to learn about the ingredients that made it most effective. What they learned was that individual clients who spontaneously referred to body awareness made the most progress in therapy. Tuning in to the *felt sense* is one of the cornerstones of the *Reversing Chronic Pain* program.

4. Experiencing the felt sense is a way of feeling more grounded, more connected with our bodies and instinctual selves. Peter Levine offers several suggestions about contacting the felt sense in *Waking the Tiger*, pp. 67–82 (Berkeley, CA: North Atlantic Books, 1997).

5. The shower pulsation exercise is presented by Dr. Levine in his audio book, *Healing Trauma* (Boulder, CO: Sounds True, 2005), p. 41.

6. My friend is Barbara Berkeley, a chiropractor in San Francisco, CA.

7. Many chronic pain clients tend to fall into two categories—either they refuse to consider medication at all *or* they overuse medication and become psychologically and/or physically dependent, believing that they cannot depend as reliably on any other treatment method. If you feel the latter is true of you, think about what you can *add* to boost the effects of your medication rather than attempting to lower or take medication away. If you are dependent or addicted and you try to reduce your medication too soon, the additional pain and fear that may result can create a setback. Adding a tool without changing your medication is a better avenue in this case because it will provide a more solid foundation on which further change can build.

8. Melzack and Wall (2004) discuss the limitations of local anesthetics due to toxic effects of more long-acting drugs (New York: Bantam, p. 225.)

9. Turk and Winter include helpful diagrams related to pacing patterns when changing pain behaviors. They suggest very short times of activity followed by much longer periods of rest. When this is successful, the next step is to lengthen activity periods followed by somewhat shorter periods of rest. See pp. 36–38 in *The Pain Survival Guide* (New York: Consumer Reports Books, 2006).

10. The Farrah Fawcett principle appears in the chapter on pain by D. Zeig and Dr. Brent Geary, (Phoenix: Milton H. Erickson Foundation Press, 2001), p. 254.

11. This exercise is based on one by Bruce Eimer in *Hypnotize Yourself Out of Pain Now!* on p. 118 (Oakland: New Harbinger, 2002).

12. Pendulation is discussed in Dr. Peter Levine's first book, *Waking the Tiger: Healing Trauma* (Berkeley, CA: North Atlantic Books, 1997), pp. 197–201, as well as in his recent book with Maggie Kline, *Trauma Through A Child's Eyes* (Berkeley, CA: North Atlantic Books, 2007).

13. "Ideodynamic healing" is a term first used by Hippolyte Bernheim in *Suggestive Therapeutics* (New York: Putnam, 1995) to refer to the impact of words as suggestions on the dynamic processes of the body. Ernest Rossi has provided a highly useful discussion of ideodynamic healing, along with techniques to encourage this process hypnotically, in his *Psychobiology of Mind-Body Healing* (New York: W.W. Norton, 1997), pp. 123–127.

CHAPTER 3

1. Research with the relaxation response is presented by Herb Benson in his book (with Marg Stark) *Timeless Healing* (New York: Simon & Schuster 1996), p. 131. Other specific benefits with chronic pain include relief of muscle aches and headaches, decrease in the intensity of pain, and increased tolerance of pain (higher pain threshold). See also Benson's 1993 article on The Relaxation Response (in Goleman & Gurin's book, *Mind-Body Medicine*, New York, Consumer Reports Books, 1993).

2. These research findings are cited by Benson in his 1993 article on p. 255.

3. Leon Chaitow discusses this need for relaxation in *Conquer Pain the Natural Way*, pp. 52–54 (San Francisco: Chronicle Books, 2002).

4. Benson views the relaxation response as opposite to the fight/flight response.

5. Eva Banyai, a well-known psychologist in Hungary, has conducted extensive research on active alert hypnosis. (See Banyai & Hilgard, *Journal of Abnormal Psychology*, 1976, pp. 218–224.) Recently, many hypnotists in the U.S. have replicated her findings, which are that active alert hypnosis has benefits equal to those achieved by formal hypnotic trance states that are marked by deep body relaxation.

6. Turk and Nash discuss these results for relaxation training with headaches in their 1993 article, "Chronic pain: New ways to cope," pp. 111–130 in Daniel Goleman & Joel Gurin (eds), *Mind-Body Medicine*, New York: Consumer Reports Books.

7. Steps in Relaxation Response training are adapted from Benson's method. See *Timeless Healing*, p. 136 (note 1 above).

8. Because nerve pain is highly traumatizing and often results from trauma to nerves, the most effective approach I've found for this is the pendulation technique first described in Chapter 2, presented here again in Chapter 3, and discussed again in depth in Chapter 8.

9. There is an enjoyable chapter on this topic in Martha Beck's *The Joy Diet* (New York: Crown, 2003). See pp. 152–177.

10. Similar suggestions in Beck's book are found on pp. 165–166.

11. Benson's review of research on the effects of faith and prayer on health concerns can be found in *Timeless Healing*, pp. 173–177.

12. For more information on kindling, see Robert Scaer's book, *The Trauma Spectrum* (New York: W.W. Norton, 2005), pp. 62–64.

13. The clenched-fist technique has been presented by many professionals as a variation of the tension-release or progressive relaxation technique. Leon Chaitow writes about this method in *Conquer Pain the Natural Way*, p. 55 (see note 3 above).

14. The "marble" technique was developed by Jordan Zarren to stimulate relaxation and as a pain distraction technique. It is explained and expanded in Bruce Eimer's book *Hypnotize Yourself Out of Pain Now!* (See pp. 56–58 and p. 110. Oakland: New Harbinger, 2002.)

CHAPTER 4

1. An excellent discussion of various applications of imagery, and the results they create, can be found in Belleruth Naparstek's book, *Invisible Heroes* (New York: Bantam, 2004), pp. 149–179.

2. Intuition as a sixth sense is presented by Christine Page in her book *Beyond the Obvious: Bringing Intuition into Our Awakening Consciousness* (London: C.W. Daniel, 2004). Other professionals, however including Pat Ogden, originator of sensorimotor therapy, believe th the sixth sense is *interoception*, resulting from the sensory nerve rece

tors that receive and transmit sensations originating from stimuli in the interior of the body. See Ogden's *Trauma and the Body* (New York: W.W. Norton, 2006), p. 15. I prefer intuition as the sixth sense.

3. Proprioceptors relay the position of various body parts, the degree of force used in various movements, and the speed and degree to which muscles are stretched.

4. Types of imagery included in *Finding the Energy to Heal* are structured and unstructured, guided, and spontaneous imagery (New York: W.W. Norton, 2000).

5. Naparstek writes in *Invisible Heroes* (see note 1 above) that imagery works down at the cellular level, where it helps stimulate the DNA into "remembering its original, miraculous blueprint" (p. 150).

6. This PET scan research was described by Martin Rossman in his article "Imagery: Learning to Use the Mind's Eye" (New York: Consumer Reports Books, 1993).

7. Post-traumatic sensitivity is discussed by Naparstek on pp. 157–160 (see note 1).

8. Eidetic imagery was developed by Ahkter Ahsen and is discussed in his book, *Psycheye* (New York: Brandon House, 1977).

9. Conflict-free Imagery is discussed in my previous book, *Finding the Energy to Heal* (see note 4) on pp. 254–256.

10. The circle of pain image is similar to the ball of pain image presented by Jeanne Achterberg and her colleagues in their book *Rituals of Healing* (New York: Bantam, 1994), p. 105.

CHAPTER 5

1. Lowen's bioenergetics model is described in his book *Bioenergetics* (New York: Penguin, 1994).

2. Darlene Cohen in *Turning Suffering Inside Out*, pp. 26–33 (Boston: Shambhala, 2000).

3. Gerald May's latest book is *The Wisdom of Wilderness* (San Francisco: Harper, 2006). His classic book is *Grace and Addiction* (San Francisco: Harper, reissue 2007).

4. Beck describes this process in *The Joy Diet*, pp. 34–42 (New York, Crown, 2003).

5. Pema Chodron's definition of mindfulness is found in her book, *The Wisdom of No Escape and the Path of Lovingkindness* (Boston: Shambhala, 1991).

6. Kabat-Zinn's research is summarized in his article on mindfulness meditation, pp. 267–269 (New York: Consumer Reports Books, 1993).

7. This discussion of the Now can be found in Tolle's *The Power of Now* (New York: New World Library, 2004) p. 33.

8. This exercise is based on the one by Tolle in *The Power of Now*, p. 41 (see above).

9. The 4-3-2-1 exercise is credited to Elizabeth Erickson, wife of Milton H. Erickson, foremost authority on modern hypnosis.

10. "Inner Strength" is a technique created by Shirley McNeal. More information on inner strength can be found in my book, *Finding the Energy to Heal*, pp. 56–57 (New York: W.W. Norton, 2000), and in Claire Frederick & Shirley McNeal's book, *Inner Strengths*, pp. 140–141 (New Jersey: Erlbaum, 1997).

11. This *metta* meditation is based on material contributed by Sharon Salzberg in her book, *The Force of Kindness* (Boulder, CO: Sounds True, 2005).

12. Larry Dossey discusses this cardiac research on prayer in his book, *Healing Words: The Power of Prayer and the Practice of Medicine* (New York: Harper Collins, 1993).

13. This quote is taken from Brother David's inspiring book, *Gratefulness, the Heart of Prayer: An Approach to Life in Fullness* (New York: Paulist Press, 1984).

14. This practice is adapted from a mindfulness approach developed by my friend, Noelle Poncelet, with whom I have taught for many years at the Esalen Institute and in the San Francisco Bay area.

CHAPTER 6

1. Some of the new methods just announced as this book goes to press are Botox injections for headache, neck, and face pain relief; short term uses of the powerful opioid drug Oxycontin; and new nutrition supplements. Always discuss these new methods with your treating professionals to decide whether they would be right for you.

2. If you are new to the world of Energy Psychology and Energy Medicine, you may want to read additional material that can help set the stage for new learning and give you more understanding of this exciting new field. This includes my second book, *Finding the Energy to Heal* (New York: W.W. Norton, 2000). Other excellent sources are *The Promise of Energy Psychology* by Feinstein, Eden, and Craig (New York: Tarcher, 2006); *Energy Diagnostics and Treatment Methods* (New York: W.W. Norton, 2000) and *Energy Tapping for Trauma* (Oakland: New Harbinger, 2007) by Fred Gallo; and *Energy Tapping* by Fred Gallo and Harry Vincenzi (Oakland: New Harbinger, 2000). These books will give you an idea of the history of energy approaches, the research that has been done and is still needed, and a more thorough overview of this approach to healing, which is largely still experimental due to the relatively small number of published, well-controlled research studies. And, because there is so much to learn all at once, and what you will learn in this chapter may be very different from anything else you have learned, you might also want to "Google" to find out more on the Internet about Energy Psychology, Energy Medicine, EFT, and meridian and chakra-based therapies, along with downloadable diagrams to help you develop confidence in finding the correct acupoints.

3. Chakra methods can be very powerful in energy healing. Since they are beyond the scope of this book, you may want to check *Creative Energies* by Dorothea Hover Kramer (New York: W.W. Norton, 2002) for possibilities in this area.

4. Catastrophizing as a form of negative thinking is discussed by Jon Kabat-Zinn in his book *Full Catastrophe Living* (New York: Delta, 1990), pp. 199–201.

5. You can learn more about the boosters and the other energy methods included in this chapter through my eight-week online course sponsored by NICABM, the National Institute for Clinical Application of Behavioral Medicine. Visit www.nicabm.com/programs for more information and registration.

6. The inner obstacles that contribute to reversals include stress, environmental toxins, food toxins, past trauma, and negative beliefs. See Feinstein, Eden, and Craig for a brief discussion (see note 1, above), pp.

36–38; and Feinstein, *Energy Psychology Interactive* (Ashland, OR: Innersource, 2004) for a more comprehensive discussion on pp. 75–92.

7. This is known as a neurolymphatic reflex point. The lymph system contains white blood cells to fight infection, and it cleanses toxins from the body. If this point is sore, it can be an indication that the lymph system is blocked in some way. Rubbing the sore spots on both sides of your chest is believed to disperse toxins and open up a flow of energy to the heart and the entire body. If there is a medical reason not to massage these points on the chest, you may rub the "karate chop" points on the sides of the hands. See Feinstein, Eden, and Craig, (note 1 above), pp. 40–42.

8. Many practitioners follow Gary Craig's Emotional Freedom Technique (EFT) "recipe" approach to affirmations, which can be found in his free, downloadable manual (see www.emofree.com). This "set-up phrase" begins with the problem first: "Even though I have this pain, I deeply and completely love and accept myself." In my practice, I prefer to lead with the positive part of the statement first. Do what's most effective for you. You might also want to consult the chapter by Gwenn Bonnell on "Pain Management: Relieving Physical and Emotional Pain" in *Freedom at Your Fingertips*, a book on the uses of EFT compiled by Ron Ball (Fredericksburg, VA: Inroads Publishing, 2006).

9. An excellent presentation by Tapas Fleming of the TAT approach can be found in Fred Gallo's *Energy Psychology in Psychotherapy: A Comprehensive Source Book* (New York: W.W. Norton, 2002), pp. 52–58.

10. I reverse steps 6 and 7 of the TAT because I have found it more powerful to focus on the personal need for forgiveness before forgiving others. Please feel free to reverse these steps back to their original order to determine which sequence works best for you.

11. If you do not get full benefits from this approach, try the following general clearing technique recommended by Tapas Fleming. For one time only, hold the pose and focus on the phrase, "I don't deserve to live, and I can't accept love, support, and healing." Then proceed through the seven steps as usual. For more information, see Fleming's book, *You Can Heal Now* (TAT International Press, 1999).

12. The eight-point protocol is the centerpiece of the Emotional Free

dom Technique (EFT) developed by Gary Craig. An excellent presentation is found in Feinstein, Eden, and Craig, Chapter 2, and at www.emofree.com.

13. The sandwich approach adds what is called "the nine-gamut treatment" after stimulating the eight points. This sequence is then followed by another round of the same eight acupoints. Although this procedure may seem somewhat strange to you at first, to try it please complete the following steps:

- *Find a spot on the back of either hand between the knuckles of your ring finger and little finger. This is called the "gamut spot." Tap, rub or touch here while completing the rest of the protocol.*
- *Close your eyes*
- *Open your eyes*
- *Without moving your head, move your eyes down to the right*
- *Then move your eyes to the left*
- *Move your eyes in a 360-degree circle in one direction*
- *Circle your eyes in the opposite direction*
- *Hum a little tune for a few seconds out loud*
- *Count out loud 1 to 5*
- *Hum your little tune again*

The "nine gamut treatment" is known as a "brain balancer." Its purpose is to stimulate a balance between left and right brain functions. For example, the experience of humming a tune is connected to the right hemisphere of the brain, while counting involves the left brain hemisphere.

To complete the sandwich, stimulate the eight points again while saying the reminder phrase "fear that my pain will increase" or "my fear." Remember to breathe at least one full breath cycle after stimulating each acupoint.

If you complete the sandwich approach and are still not getting good results, you may need to use energy (muscle) testing to pinpoint reminder phrases, check for reversals, and evaluate results. Information on muscle testing can be downloaded from Gary Craig's website, www.emofree.com. Another good resource for energy testing and energy approaches with pain is *The Top Ten Pain Releasers* by Arlene Green (Chapel Hill, NC: Green Angel Press, 1993).

14. EMDR was developed by Francine Shapiro and first piloted with Vietnam veterans and women who had been raped. The model has since been expanded to address complex past trauma as well as various symptoms related to trauma including depression, anxiety, panic, and pain. One good resource for nonprofessionals who want to learn about EMDR is *EMDR* (New York: Basic Books, 1997) by Francine Shapiro and Margot Silk-Forrest. Readers who are professionals trained in EMDR may want to refer to Laurel Parnell's book, *A Therapist's Guide to EMDR* (New York: W.W. Norton, 2007). You may also want to refer to Mark Grant's website: www.overcomingpain.com.

15. The butterfly hug was created by students of John Hartung and Michael Galvin, who are well-known for combining Energy Psychology methods with EMDR. You can read about their work in their book *Energy Psychology and EMDR: Combining Forces to Optimize Treatment* (New York: W.W. Norton, 2003).

16. WHEE also stands for "Wholistic Hybrid derived from EMDR and EFT" and was developed by Daniel Benor. To find out more about WHEE, visit Dr. Benor's website at http://wholistichealingresearch.com for additional information, research studies, and modifications.

17. The "three thumps" popularized by Donna Eden can be found in her book *Energy Medicine*, pp. 63–68 (New York: Tarcher/Putnam, 1998).

CHAPTER 7

1. For more information about the Egoscue method, see his book *Pain Free* (New York: Bantam, 1998).

2. A good basic book on stretching is *Stretching* by Bob Anderson. He lists these benefits for stretching on page 11 (Bolinas, CA: Shelter Publications, 2000).

3. An excellent book on trigger point therapy self-treatment is available by Clair Davies and colleagues: *The Trigger Point Therapy Workbook* (Oakland: New Harbinger, 2004).

4. For research on the benefits of acupuncture, visit the following web site: http:odp.od.nih.gov/consenses/cons/107/107_intro.htm.

CHAPTER 8

1. To read more about the biology of trauma, consult Robert Scaer's book, *The Trauma Spectrum* (New York: WW Norton, 2005).
2. Belleruth Naparstek discusses the connection between childhood trauma and chronic pain on pp. 78–80 of her book *Invisible Heroes* (New York: Bantam, 2004). I also discuss this topic in my article, "Hypnosis with Depression, Posttraumatic Stress Disorder, and Chronic Pain" in Michael Yapko's book, *Hypnosis and Treating Depression* (New York: Routledge, 2006), pp. 218–220.
3. For excellent information on the biology of traumatic dissociation, see Robert Scaer, *The Trauma Spectrum*, pp. 177–204 (see note 1). For a more general discussion of dissociation, see my first book, *Healing the Divided Self* (New York: W.W. Norton, 1995), pp. 17–18, and 179–198.
4. Somatic Experiencing is presented in Dr. Peter Levine's books, *Waking the Tiger, and Trauma Through A Child's Eyes* (the latter co-written with Maggie Kline), as well as in Dr. Levine's audio books published by Sounds True. (See chapter 2, note 5, for publisher data).
5. Pendulation is similar to bilateral stimulation used in EMDR (Eye Movement Desensitization and Reprocessing) yet there are important differences. While both methods promote the stimulation of right and left brain functions, pendulation is designed to rebalance nervous system activation, while the purpose of EMDR is to assist in trauma reprocessing at cognitive levels as well as with body experience.
6. The dissociative table technique was originally developed by George Fraser, MD, and can be downloaded at https://scholarsbank.uoregon.edu/dspace/bitstream/1794/1467/1/Diss_4_4_7_OCR.pdf. Further suggestions for developing the "inner table" technique can be found in Bruce Eimer's *Hypnotize Yourself Out of Pain Now!* (Oakland: New Harbinger, 2002), pp. 181–187, and in Jack and Helen Watkins, *Ego States* (New York, W.W. Norton, 1997), pp. 108–116.

CHAPTER 9

1. Belleruth Naparstek discusses this research on the impact of trauma in *Invisible Heroes*, pp. 51–55 (New York, Bantam, 2004).

2. Steven Levine's book is *Unattended Sorrow* (New York: Rodale, 2005).

3. This definition of grief is found in *Unattended Sorrow*, p. 10.

4. Finding a trained professional to work with may also feel challenging if you have never worked with a psychotherapist or have had less than positive experiences in the past. Consult the resources section in Appendix 2 for help.

5. This script is based on one presented by Bruce Eimer in *Hypnotize Yourself Out of Pain Now!* pp. 152–154 (Oakland: New Harbinger, 2002).

6. This meditation is based on ones created by Belleruth Naparstek in *Invisible Heroes*, pp. 215–220 (see note 1).

7. Janis Abram Spring, *How Can I Forgive You?* (New York: HarperCollins, 2004), pp. 53–54.

8. The Door of Forgiveness exercise was created by Helen Watkins. See Watkins and Watkins, *Ego States*, pp. 133–134 (New York: W.W. Norton, 1997).

9. Fred Gallo's midline energy technique (MET) can be found in *Energy Diagnostic and Treatment Methods* (New York: W.W. Norton, 2000), pp. 132–134. Dr. Gallo named this technique NAEM (Negative Affect Erasing Method). I prefer to call it the midline technique.

CHAPTER 10

1. There are many, many powerful paths to healing not included in this book. One excellent resource is my book *Finding the Energy to Heal* (New York: W.W. Norton, 2000), which will give you an idea of the potential of many different methods included in this book as well as how to combine methods for more lasting results. Another excellent reference is chapter 14 in Belleruth Naparstek's book, *Invisible Heroes* (New York: Bantam, 2004), pp. 289–321. Here she reviews what she calls imagery-based therapies, which include EMDR, Somatic Experiencing, EFT and TFT, as well as methods not covered in this book such as TIR (Traumatic Incident Reduction).

References

Achterberg, Jeanne, Dossey, Barbara, and Kolkmeier, Leslie (1994). *Rituals of Healing: Using Imagery for Health and Wellness*. New York: Bantam.

Ahsen, Akter (1977). *Psycheye: Self-analytic Consciousness*. New York: Brandon House.

Anderson, Robert (2000). *Stretching: 20th Anniversary Revised Edition*. Bolinas, CA: Shelter Publications.

Banyai, Eva, and Hilgard, Ernest (1976). "A comparison of active-alert hypnotic induction with traditional relaxation induction." *Journal of Abnormal Psychology* 85: 218–224.

Beck, Martha (2003). *The Joy Diet: 10 Daily Practices for a Happier Life*. New York: Crown.

Benson, Herb (1993). "The Relaxation Response," pp. 233–258 in Daniel Goleman and Joel Gurin, *Mind-Body Medicine: How to Use Your Mind for Better Health*. New York: Consumer Reports Books.

Benson, Herb, and Klipper, Miriam (2000). *The Relaxation Response*. New York: Wholecare.

Benson, Herb, and Stark, Marg (1996). *Timeless Healing: The Power and Biology of Belief*. New York: Simon & Schuster.

Caudill, Margaret (2002). *Managing Pain Before It Manages You*. New York: Guilford.

Chaitow, Leon (2002). *Conquer Pain the Natural Way: A Practical Guide*. San Francisco: Chronicle Books.

Challem, Jack (2003). *The Inflammation Syndrome*. New York: Wiley.

Chodron, Pema (1991). *The Wisdom of No Escape and the Path of Lovingkindness*. Boston: Shambhala.

Cohen, Darlene (2000). *Turning Suffering Inside Out: A Zen Approach to Living with Physical and Emotional Pain*. Boston: Shambhala.

Davies, Clair, Davies, Amber, and Simons, David (2004). *The Trigger Point Therapy Workbook: Your Self-Treatment Guide for Pain Relief*, 2nd Ed. Oakland, CA: New Harbinger.

Dillard, James (2002). *The Chronic Pain Solution: Your Personal Path to Pain Relief*. New York: Bantam.

Dossey, Larry (1993). *Healing Words: The Power of Prayer and the Practice of Medicine*. New York: Harper Collins.

Eden, Donna (1998). *Energy Medicine*. New York: Tarcher/Putnam.

Egoscue, Pete (1998). *Pain Free: A Revolutionary Method for Stopping Chronic Pain*. New York: Bantam.

Eimer, Bruce (2002). *Hypnotize Yourself Out of Pain Now*. Oakland, CA: New Harbinger.

Feinstein, David (2004). *Energy Psychology Interactive: Rapid Interventions for Lasting Change*. Ashland, OR: Innersource.

Feinstein, David, Eden, Donna, and Craig, Gary (2006). *The Promise of Energy Psychology: Revolutionary Tools for Dramatic Personal Change*. New York: Tarcher.

Fleming, Tapas (2002). "The Tapas Acupressure Technique," pp. 52–58 in Fred Gallo (ed.), *Energy Psychology in Psychotherapy*. New York: Norton.

Fleming, Tapas (1999). *You Can Heal Now: The Tapas Acupressure Technique*. Redondo Beach, CA: TAT International Press.

Frederick, Claire, and McNeal, Shirley (1997). *Inner Strengths: Contemporary Psychotherapy and Hypnosis for Ego-Strengthening*. New Jersey: Erlbaum.

Gallo, Fred. (2007). */Energy Tapping for Trauma: Rapid Relief from Post-Traumatic Stress Using Energy Psychology*. /Oakland, CA: New Harbinger.

Gallo, Fred (ed.) (2002). *Energy Psychology in Psychotherapy*. New York: Norton.

Gallo, Fred (2000). *Energy Diagnostic and Treatment Methods*. New York: Norton.

Gendlin, Eugene (1982). *Focusing*. New York: Bantam.

Gladwell, Malcolm (2002). *The Tipping Point: How Little Things Can Make A Big Difference*. New York: Little, Brown, and Company.

Goleman, Daniel, and Gurin, Joel (eds.) (1993) *Mind-Body Medicine: How to Use Your Mind for Better Health*, New York: Consumer Reports Books.

Kabat-Zinn, Jon (1993). "Mindfulness meditation: Health benefits of an

ancient Buddhist practice," pp. 259–275 in Daniel Goleman and Joel Gurin (eds.), *Mind-Body Medicine: How to Use Your Mind for Better Health*. New York: Consumer Reports Books.

Kabat-Zinn, Jon (1990). *Full Catastrophe Living: Using the Wisdom of Your Body and Mind to Face Stress, Pain, and Illness*. New York: Delta.

Levine, Peter (2005). *Healing Trauma: A Pioneering Program for Restoring the Wisdom of Your Body*. Boulder, CO: Sounds True (audio program).

Levine, Peter (1997). *Waking the Tiger: Healing Trauma*. Berkeley, CA: North Atlantic Books.

Levine, Peter, and Kline, Maggie (2007). *Trauma Through A Child's Eyes*. Berkeley, CA: North Atlantic Books.

Levine, Stephen (2005). *Unattended Sorrow: Recovering from Loss and Reviving the Heart*. New York: Rodale.

Lowen, Alexander (1994). *Bioenergetics*. New York: Penguin.

May, Gerald (reissue 2007). *Grace and Addiction: Love and Spirituality in the Healing of Addictions*. San Francisco: Harper.

May, Gerald (2006). *The Wisdom of Wilderness: Experiencing the Healing Powers of Nature*. San Francisco: Harper.

Melzack, Ronald, and Wall, Patrick (2004). *The Challenge of Pain. 2nd Edition*. New York: Bantam.

Naparstek, Belleruth (2004). *Invisible Heroes: Survivors of Trauma and How They Heal*. New York: Bantam.

Ogden, Pat, Minton, Kekuni, and Pain, Clare (2006). *Trauma and the Body: A Sensorimotor Approach to Psychotherapy*. New York: Norton.

Page, Christine (2004). *Beyond the Obvious: Bringing Intuition into our Awakening Consciousness*. London: C.W. Daniel Company, Ltd.

Pert, Candace (2002). *The Molecules of Emotion: Why You Feel the Way You Feel*. New York: Scribner.

Phillips, Maggie (2006). "Hypnosis with depression, posttraumatic stress disorder, and chronic pain," pp. 217–241 in Michael Yapko (ed.), *Hypnosis and Treating Depression: Applications in Clinical Practice*. New York: Routledge.

Phillips, Maggie (2000). *Finding the Energy to Heal: How EMDR, Hypnosis, TFT, Imagery, and Body-Focused Therapy Help Restore Mindbody Health*. New York: Norton.

Phillips, Maggie, and Frederick, Claire (1995). *Healing the Divided Self: Clinical and Ericksonian Hypnotherapy for Post-traumatic and Dissociative Conditions*. New York: Norton.

Rossi, Ernest (1997). *The Psychobiology of Mindbody Healing: New Concepts of Therapeutic Hypnosis*. New York: Norton.

Rossman, Martin (1993). "Imagery: How to Use the Mind's Eye," pp. 291–300 in Daniel Goleman and Joel Gurin (eds.), *Mind-Body Medicine: How to Use Your Mind for Better Health*, New York: Consumer Reports Books.

Salzberg, Sharon (2005). *The Force of Kindness: Change Your Life with Love & Compassion*. Boulder, CO: Sounds True. (audio program)

Scaer, Robert (2005). *The Trauma Spectrum: Hidden Wounds and Human Resiliency*. New York: Norton.

Spring, Janis Abram (2004). *How Can I Forgive You? The Courage to Forgive, the Freedom Not To*. New York: HarperCollins.

Tolle, Eckhard (2004). *The Power of Now: A Guide to Spiritual Enlightenment*. New York: New World Library.

Turk, Dennis, and Nash, Justin (1993). "Chronic pain: New ways to cope," pp. 111–130 in Daniel Goleman & Joel Gurin (eds), *Mind-Body Medicine*, New York: Consumer Reports Books.

Turk, Dennis, and Winter, Frits (2006). *The Pain Survival Guide: How to Reclaim Your Life*. Washington, DC: American Psychological Association.

Watkins, John, and Watkins, Helen (1997). *Ego States: Theory and Therapy*. New York: Norton.

Zeig, Jeffrey, and Geary, B. (2001). "Ericksonian approaches to pain management," pp. 252–262 in Geary & Zeig (eds.), *The Handbook of Ericksonian Psychotherapy*. Phoenix, AZ: The Milton H. Erickson Foundation Press.

Index

A

Acceptance, 175–76

Active alert hypnosis, 46, 205

Acupressure, 142

Acupuncture, 105, 142, 212

Acute pain, 4

Adrenaline, 146

Affirmations, 111–13, 125, 135, 159, 210

"AIDS cocktail" approach, 12, 106, 202

Amygdala, 4, 148–49

Anderson, Bob, 133

Anger, 165. See also Emotional pain

Antioxidants, 16

Anxiety, 47–48, 150–51

Attention, 89

Attitude
of openness, 30
toward pain, 27

Autoimmune disorders, 149

B

B-complex vitamins, 195

Beck, Martha, 88

Beginner's mind, 89

Benson, Herb, 45, 46, 51, 57, 100

Bioenergetics, 86, 207

Biofeedback, 203

Body
feedback from, 57–58
finding a sanctuary within, 23
-focused therapy, 33
-mind connection, 1–2, 90
sensations, 30–31
trusting wisdom of, 193

Body awareness. See also Body awareness skills
attitude and, 30
definition of, xxii
importance of, xviii

Body awareness skills
breathing, 20–23
building on success, 194
energizing, 123–25
feeling, 39–41
imagining, 80–82
loving, 177–79
mindful meditation, 102–3
moving, 143–44
pendulating, 161–63
relaxing, 61–62
review of, 181–87

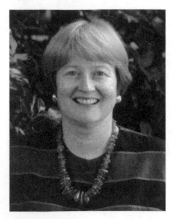

About the Author

A licensed psychologist with thirty years of experience in clinical practice, Maggie Phillips, PhD, leads workshops, online seminars, and teleclasses nationally and internationally on chronic pain, hypnosis, Somatic Experiencing,® stress disorders, the treatment of trauma, and uses of energy psychology and other approaches in mindbody healing. In her private practice, she specializes in the treatment of complex chronic emotional and physical pain, and post-traumatic and dissociative stress conditions.

Dr. Phillips is the author of two previous books as well as numerous articles and book chapters. She has been honored with the Cornelia Wilbur Award from the International Society for the Study of Dissociation (ISSD) for her contributions to the field of trauma and dissociation, the Crasilneck Award for excellence in writing, and the President's Award from the American Society of Clinical Hypnosis. In addition, she is contributing editor for the *American Journal of Clinical Hypnosis*.

A frequent presenter at conferences around the world, Dr. Phillips has been awarded Fellow status in both the American Society of Clinical Hypnosis (ASCH) and in the International Society for the Study of Dissociation (ISSD). She lives in Oakland, California.